Addiction
A Misdiagnosis

Reward Deficiency Syndrome
Diagnosis & Treatment

James V. Potter, Ph.D. & Paula M. Potter, MA

ADDICTION: A MISDIAGNOSIS

REWARD DEFICIENCY SYNDROME
DIAGNOSIS AND TREATMENT

ISBN-10: 1540628191   ISBN-13: 978-1540628190

Unless otherwise noted, all Biblical Scripture quotations in this volume are from the New International Version, Student Edition (NIV Study Bible), copyright ©1985, Zondervan Corporation, Grand Rapids, Michigan, USA

ISBN-10: 1540628191   ISBN-13: 978-1540628190

Publishers ~   Advocare Publishing Co.
              Redding, California USA

Printers ~   CreateSpace

Printed in the United States of America

Preface

Dr. James Potter, and his wife Paula, are both Licensed and Ordained Ministers of the Gospel, Licensed Clinical Pastoral-Counselors, Certified Domestic Violence Specialists, Addiction Rehabilitation Specialists and Prepare/Enrich Counselors and Trainers. Dr. James Potter, and his wife, Paula Potter, are both adjunct faculty members for Vision International University and Advocare Institute.

Dr. Potter and Paula are Cofounders and Trustees of Jubilee Enterprises, Founders and Directors of Advocare Family Skills Institute and Advocare Publishing Co. Dr. Potter is Past President of Agape Family Services, Inc., and Alliance Recovery Services, in California; President of Special People Hawaii, an Employee Assistance Program consulting firm in Hawaii; Past-president of Victory Family Care Centers, a multidisciplinary counseling ministry in Hawaii.

Dr. Potter is a member of the World Association of Online Educators, mentoring students world wide. He has served on the Board of Family Care Services International, the Advisory Board of the American Association of Family Counselors, and the American Institute of Counseling. He is past president of the International Christian Counselor's Association and past International Director of the National Christian Counselor's Association.

Dr. Potter served as a Gubernatorial appointed member of the Hawaii Area Service Board on Mental Health and Substance Abuse from 1991 through 1994, and Coordinator for the Hawaii Chapter of CAPS [Christian Association for Psychological Studies] in 1994 and 1995.

Dr. Potter is listed in numerous editions of: "Who's

Who in Religion," "Who's Who in America," "Who's Who in Education," and "Who's Who in the World," Marquis Who's Who's Publications Board. Potter was the recipient of the American Biographical Institute "Man of the Year" award and the International Biographical Centre's "Men of Achievement" award, in 1993. Potter was recognized as a Fellow of the American College of Forensic Counselors in 2001.

Dr. Potter and Paula have served in the office of pastors, associate pastors and evangelists, and pastoral counselors within local churches for many years. They have conducted seminars and workshops in *Prayer, Couple Communication & Conflict Resolution, Anger Management & The Prevention of Family Violence, Successful Parenting, Substance Abuse Prevention and Treatment, and Spiritual Growth* throughout the Hawaiian Islands and several western states. Dr. Potter is also a national presenter in the areas of Domestic Violence Prevention and Abatement and Substance Abuse and Addiction Prevention and Treatment.

Dedication

This book is dedicated to the tens of millions of men and women worldwide who have been misdiagnosed as having the disease of addiction, and have lived their lives under the stigma of being identified as an addict.

We include in this dedication those millions of individuals who have spent years behind bars for crimes committed while under the influence of a mind-altering substance or activity; whose lives have been destroyed by being convicted and incarcerated for having a disease.

May this small book, and the recent contribution of many other authors on this topic serve to commence the repatriation of those who have lost their freedoms, their right to vote, their families, professions and so much more due to their being misdiagnosed as an addict, which is claimed to be incurable; rather than being treated for the curable disease of Reward Deficiency Syndrome.

Contents

Chapter One
Don't Call Me Addict

Consider how you would feel if you were afflicted with diabetes or say anemia or epilepsy, and instead of calling you by your given name, people referred to you as "the cancer," "the anemic," or "the 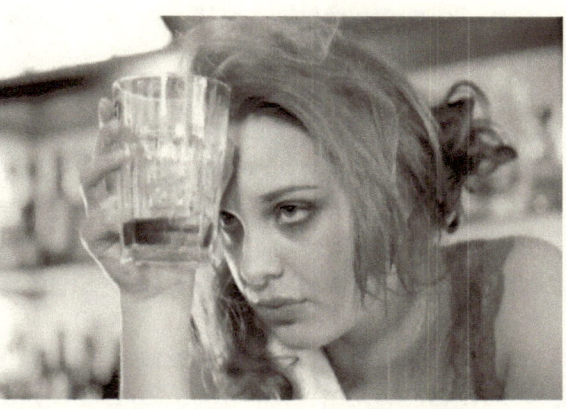 epileptic." No one calls another these names because we intuitively understand that to do so would be very insensitive and disrespectful; yet, we think nothing of calling someone "a substance abuser," or "an addict."

I can imagine many of you thinking, 'yes, but there's a big difference: substance abuse and addiction – unlike cancer, anemia and epilepsy – are self-imposed, brought on by one's own lifestyle. This, however, is faulty thinking. The onset of Diabetes, Type II is brought on by ones lifestyle, as is COPD but we don't refer to the individual suffering from these diseases as "the diabetic," or "the emphysematous."

Normally, when we consider it necessary to make reference to someone's disease or disability we employ an empathic statement such as, my sister who has diabetes, or my brother who suffers from epilepsy, or seizures. It is doubtful that we would identify them by their disability, disease, mental or physical challenge. We normally call others by their given name and use it to identify them when speaking about them to a third party.

Why then are we so inconsiderate when we are dealing with those suffering from a chemical dependency or an activity addiction such as compulsive gambling? Even tough these diseases are self-inflicted, when one's disease or disorder has resulted in their homelessness, or their incarceration, they are still a human being – not an "it" or an "other."

Not a single one of us is perfect; we all suffer from the effect of sin – the most pervasive self-inflicted illness there is. Moreover, this disease is fatal. As the apostle Paul stated in his letter to the church at Rome, *"The wages of sin is death"* (Rom 6:23).

I Doc Potter] don't know what you have personally struggled with, perhaps are still striving to overcome; but whatever it is, you are still a human being, still a child of God. What if every person you met glared at you, pointed their finger at you and called you 'sinner, sinner'? How would that make you feel? How likely is it that you would let those who addressed you in this manner, speak into your life?

No doubt, you would be offended, reticent to embrace anything they said or accept their help, if offered – and rightly so. But, this is precisely what the 12-Step recovery programs have done, and continue to do. In fact, they pretty much demand that everyone attending one of their meetings label themselves with the 'appropriate' self-deprecating title of alcoholic, drug addict, overeater, etc., etc.

Jesus, addressing the Jewish Torah teachers, said, *"For the mouth speaks what overflows from the heart. The good person brings forth good things from his store of good, and the evil person brings forth evil things from his store of evil. Moreover, I tell you this: on the Day of Judgment people will have to give account for every careless word they have spoken; for by your own words*

2

you will be acquitted, and by your own words you will be condemned" (Matt 12:34-37 CJB).

Consider the harmful consequence of *this in light of the words of King Solomon, who wrote: "A fool's mouth is his undoing, and his lips are a snare to his soul. . . . Death and life are in the power of the tongue: and they that love it shall eat the fruit thereof"* (Pro 18:7 &21). *"For as the thoughts of a man's heart are, so is he"* (Pro 23:7).

The perfect rehabilitation program must be based on absolute truth; and the unquestionable, undeniable truth is that every man, woman and child is a child of God, created by Him and for His pleasure.

There are no addicts for God did not create addicts. There are, however, many children of God who have become addicted to many, many things, most of which impair one's optimum functionality and have life-damaging consequences. To avert these consequences, one must alter their lifestyle, restoring the creation model of Imago Dei [the image of God].

No doubt most who are reading this book have read – or heard – the words found in Genesis – the Book of Beginnings – concerning the origin of man. *"God said, "Let us make humankind in our image, in the likeness of ourselves; and let them rule over the fish in the sea, the birds in the air, the animals, and over all the earth, and over every crawling creature that crawls on the earth." So God created humankind in his own image; in the image of God he created him: male and female he created them"* (Gen 1:26-27 CJB).

While most have, no doubt, read or heard these words many times, few have taken time to meditate on them in order to discover the origin of this phenomenon we refer to as addiction. Unquestionably, Psychologist Carl Jung came close when he penned these words, that "*all*

3

addictions are mankind's maladaptive attempts to find God."

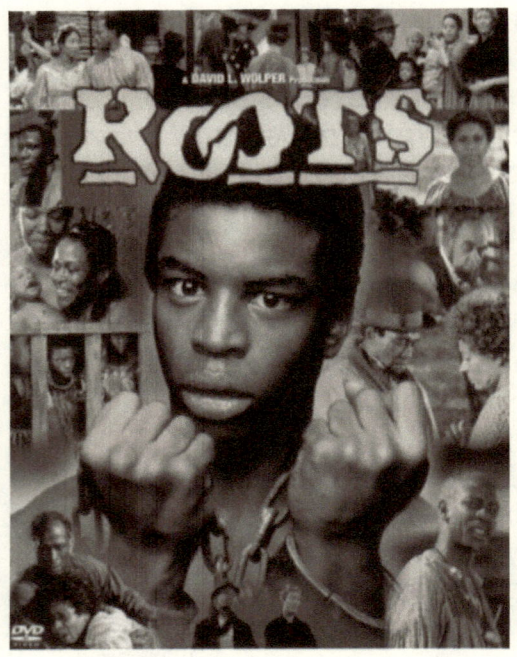

Mankind seems driven to discover his roots or heritage. In the nearly thirty years of our counseling ministry virtually every adopted person we have counseled has either been, or currently is, on a quest to discover their true identity. Children know intuitively that their identity stems from that of their parents, and seem to understand that they can never know themselves until they know who gave them life. They may never have met either birth parent, yet they are dependent upon them.

This dependency is even more apparent in the relationship between Elohim [the Divine Ones, or Godhead] and mankind. Man was made in God's image, stemming from a Hebrew root word meaning an illusionary phantom, shadow or mirror image. He was also created in the likeness of Elohim, a term stemming from a Hebrew word meaning resemblance or similitude.

A mirror image or shadow is dependent upon the substantive model it is reflecting; without that model the image or likeness cannot, does not, exist. We are, therefore, wholly de pendent upon God. Our nature is that of a dependent being – the essence of which can never endure independently.

God is the source of all light. From Him all light emanates (Gen 1:4). He is the light of the world (Jn 9:5); Without Him, there is naught but darkness. God is life and the source thereof (Job 33:4; Jn 5:26). Separated from God there is naught but death (Jn 8:12).

Separated by his/her rebellion, from Elohim, the substance of whom he is but an illusionary reflection, mankind's nature was still that of a dependent being. And since, in his state of rebellion he choose to defy God, he turned his 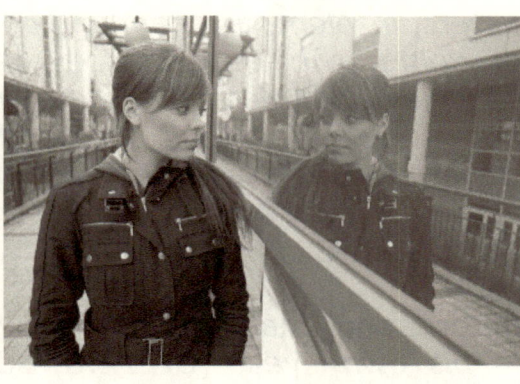 dependency elsewhere. This is described by the apostle Paul in his letter to the Church of Rome.

"For although they knew God, they neither glorified him as God nor gave thanks to him, but their thinking became futile and their foolish hearts were darkened. Although they claimed to be wise, they became fools and exchanged the glory of the immortal God for images made to look like mortal man and birds and animals and reptiles. Therefore God gave them over in the sinful desires of their hearts to sexual impurity for the degrading of their bodies with one another. They exchanged the truth of God for a lie, and worshiped and served created things rather than the Creator –who is forever praised. Amen.

"Because of this, God gave them over to shameful lusts. Even their women exchanged natural relations for unnatural ones. In the same way the men also abandoned natural relations with women and were inflamed with lust for one another. Men committed indecent acts with other men, and received in themselves the due penalty for their perversion.

"Furthermore, since they did not think it worthwhile to retain the knowledge of God, he gave them over to a depraved mind, to do what ought not to be done. They have become filled with every kind of wickedness, evil, greed and depravity. They are full of envy, murder, strife, deceit and malice. They are gossips, slanderers, God-haters, insolent, arrogant and boastful; they invent ways of doing evil; they disobey their parents; they are senseless, faithless, heartless, ruthless. Although they know God's righteous decree that those who do such things deserve death, they not only continue to do these very things but also approve of those who practice them" (Rom 1:21-32).

Before long, man was *"doing whatsoever seemed right in his own eyes"* (Dt 12:8; Jdg 17:26; 21:25). Still dependent, still feeling called to worship a being higher than themselves, they began worshipping the stars, the moon and the sun.

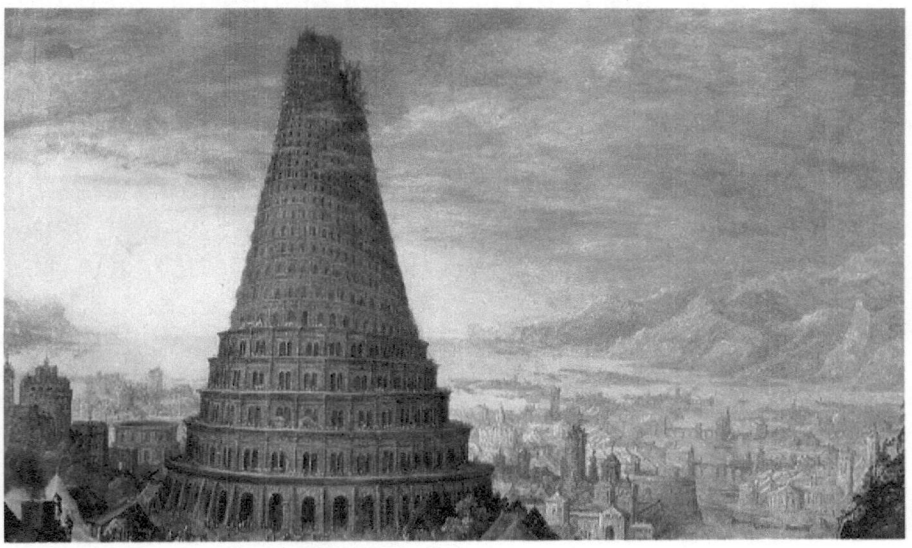

Obsessed with the idea to worship a seen deity they began creating idols of wood, stone and precious metals. Eventually they even worshipped animals, demons and even themselves.

Nothing that they tried satisfied their need. In desperation they allowed their obsessions to take them lower and lower. Over time they spiraled lower and lower until they became known as children of the devil (1 Jn 3:10). They had become what we today call addicts – ever seeking, but never satisfied.

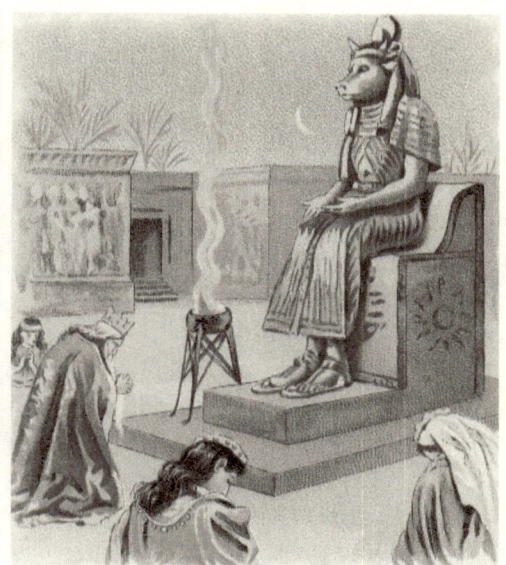

Chapter Two
The History of Addiction

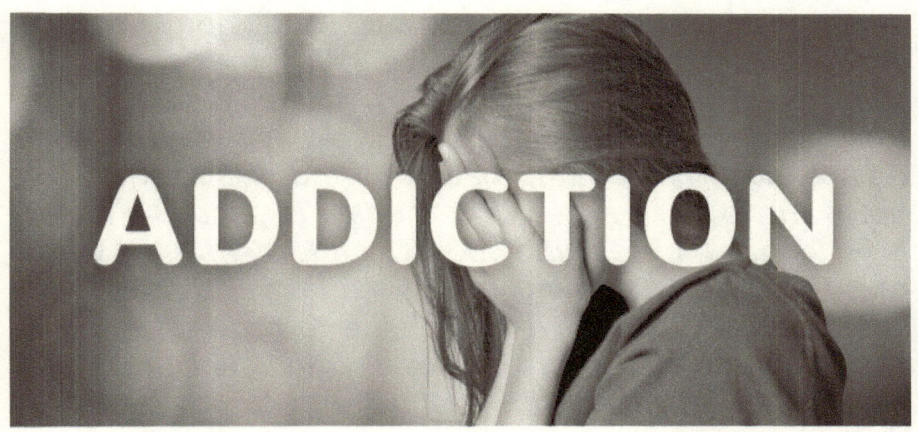

Addictions are not a 21st. century phenomena. Ancient Chinese writings dating back at to about 3,000 B.C. describe the abuse of alcohol and drugs. The Judeo-Christian Bible, more widely known in the Western world, also has a great deal to say on the subject of addictions. For example, King Solomon ̶writing during the tenth century B.C. advised us that "Wine is a mocker   *and beer a brawler; whoever is led astray by them is not wise"* (Pro 20:1).

Solomon then goes on to tell us the outcome of one who allows himself or herself to be thus led astray: He asks, *"Who has woe? Who without cause? Who has bloodshot eyes."* The answer he gives, reveals the chain of addiction. *"Those who linger over wine, those who go in to sample bowls of mixed drink. Do not,"* he warns, *"gaze at wine when it is red, when it sparkles in the cup; when it goes down smoothly! In the end, it bites like a snake and poisons like a viper. Your eyes will see strange sights and your mind imagine strange things. You will be like one sleeping on the high seas, lying atop of the rigging.*

"They hit me," you will say, "but I'm not hurt! they beat me up, but I don't feel it. Oh, when will I wake up so I can find another drink?" (Proverbs 23:29-35).

The New Testament apostle, Paul, demonstrated his understanding of the dilemma of addiction when he penned Romans 7: 14-20. *"We know that the law is spiritual, but I am carnal (fleshly), sold as a slave to sin. I do not understand what I do. For what I want to do, 1 do not, but what I hate, that I do. And, if I do what I do not want to do, I agree that the law is good. As it is, it is no longer I myself who does it, but it is sin living within me. I know that nothing good lives in me, that is in my sinful nature, for I have the desire to do what is good, but I cannot carry it out. For what I do is not the good I want to do; no, the evil I do not want to do, I keep on doing."*

"So then," he continues, *"I find this law at work: when I want to do good, evil is right there with me. For in my inner-being I delight in God's law; but I see another law at work in the members of my body, waging war against the law of my mind and making me a prisoner of the law if sin at work in my members. What a wretched man I am,"* he cries, *"Who will rescue me from this body of death?"*

Is addiction, as some claim, just a sin (a moral issue); a problem behavior (just a bad habit); the product of mental weakness? Or is it a physical disease as those involved in 12-Step groups such as AA, NA, etc., would have us believe? The answer to each of these alternative origins is an unequivocal yes, yes, yes – and yes. However, addiction is even more than the combination of them all!

Addiction is unquestionably a disease – a disease of the body, mind (soul) and spirit; a disease that is chronic, progressive, and fatal if left untreated.

But, if a disease, a disease of what" That is where is this disease located? If one suffers from diabetes we know that they have a disease within the pancreas; if one suffers from astigmatism or glaucoma we know that they have a disorder within 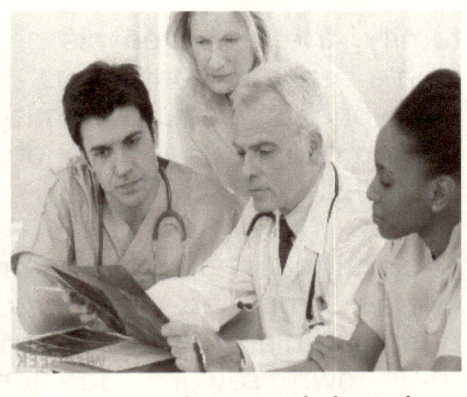 the eye, and if one has cirrhosis, we understand that they have a diseased liver. But, where is this so called "disease" of alcoholism located?

It is a disease that affects every aspect of what it means to be fully human —debilitating one's spirit, mind, emotions, body, relationships, environment, etc. According to current research, this disease is centered in the brain. Addiction —that is, the propensity toward addiction —is centered in the pain-pleasure center (or reward pathway) within mankind's brain. It is a disease that is rapidly becoming known as something far more descriptive, being renamed by leading experts as "The

Reward Deficiency Syndrome."
The history of the origin of addiction is far to complicated to cover in detail in this volume. For those desiring to pursue this, we recommend our book, "Counseling Addicts and Offenders, J.V. & P.M. Potter, Advocare Publishing Co., Redding, California. In that volume we examine the sociological and legal history contributing to this worldwide malady. This volume, in contrast is dedicated to understanding the Reward Deficiency Syndrome and setting forth a biopsychosociospiritual approach to addiction rehabilitation and recovery.

Addiction is a disease that affects not only the individual abusing alcohol drugs, food or some activity such as gambling or pornography; it impacts that individual's family, friends, even his or her environment. Addiction is in a sense a "contagious" disease in that it traumatizes everyone in close proximity and relationship with the person caught up in their obsessive-compulsive behavior patterns.

The traumatized family members – those who are close to one struggling with addiction – are exposed to their brain chemistry, which contributes to the development of their own reward deficiency syndrome. Commonly referred to as codependency, or co-addiction, it meets all the criteria of a disease – being chronic, progressive and if left untreated, fatal.

In recognition of the long established disease concept of addiction and co-addiction or codependency, the current ongoing research findings relevant to the reward deficiency syndrome, the failure of the "war on drugs" to significantly reduce the abuse of illicit substances, and the resulting rise in the incidence of these diseases, it is apparent that this battle must be fought in a different manner.

In recognition of this, we turn now to examine several alternative battle plans and their implementation.

Chapter Three
The War Against Addiction

It is past time that we reexamine the failure that has been titled, "The War on Drugs." During the past four decades, the US alone has spent more than a trillion dollars ($1,000,000,000,000) on this war and failed miserably.

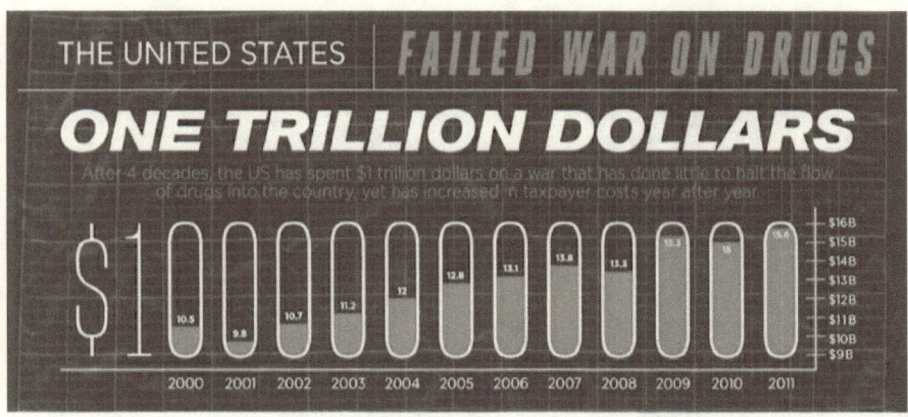

Attacking the supply side of illicit substances has done little other than increase the selling price. Hardly a deterrent for the criminal-minded producer, courier or dealer! Moreover, addictions such as pornography and gambling now represent a greater drain on society than chemical abuse and dependency. If we are to become victorious in this war, it is time that we focus our resources on increasing the effectiveness of prevention, as well as providing effective treatment for those to whom prevention has come too late.

One greatly needed weapon in this "war against addiction" is the development of more accurate assessments —assessments that determine one's propensity to addiction; the substances and activities one is vulnerable to; as well as the damage already done by their involvement in these.

Another need is informed treatment planning – based on scientifically determined information rather than "best guess" methodologies that have been relied on in the past. In order to realize improved treatment outcomes, appropriate methodologies must be developed that attend to the varied aspects of the disease in an fitting manner and an acceptable order.

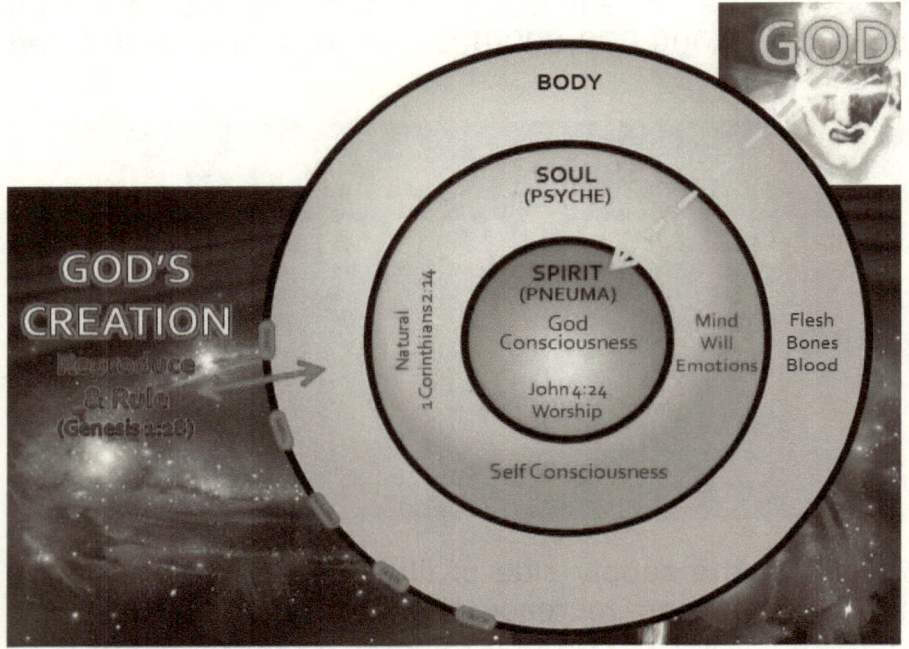

Since the disease of addiction is one of body, soul (or mind) and spirit, appropriate interventions must address all three domains, and address them in the appropriate order. Secularly focused programs often address spiritual issues in such a vague, lackadaisical manner that spiritual healing languishes. In contrast, many faith-based programs so prematurely address and over emphasize the spiritual aspects of recovery that the healing of body and mind (soul) languish.

Addiction, as Jellinek pointed out decades ago, is a progressive/regressive disease. That is, the further the disease progresses, the further the emotional and motivational age of the person regresses. The disease affects one's entire being – first the spirit, then the soul (or mind), and finally the body. It would seem both logical and appropriate then, that healing should address each of these disorders, but in the reverse, alleviating first the physical manifestations and problems, then the psychological distress and faulty thinking, and lastly the spiritual despair resulting from one's alienation from a Higher Power (God), and from authority in general.

The Jellinek Curve

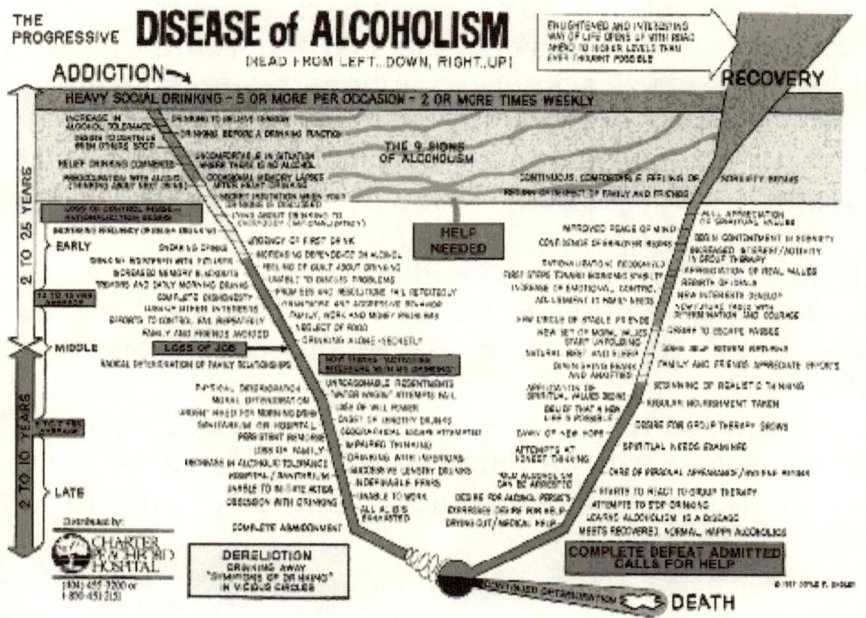

To attempt spiritual restoration initially, frequently results in the individual's premature termination of treatment and a return to their drug or activity of choice, relied on to ameliorate their increased guilt and shame, and assuage their physical and/or psychological pain. And, a psychological only approach often fails when life-management skill-training precedes physical restoration and/or when recovery is terminated without addressing the restoration of the human spirit.

The term "recovery" is in the truest sense a misnomer since most individuals suffering from an addiction have never enjoyed a period in life that was filled with emotional and environmental peace and tranquillity. They have never tasted that sense of well-being that other people enjoy. And, they have never achieved maturity. Instead, most suffer from moderate to severe arrested development.

Most individuals suffering from one or multiple addictions have – according to current research – some genetic/biological predisposition to the reward deficiency syndrome. The others develop said syndrome as a result of early life physical injury, emotional trauma of sufficient intensity and/or duration to create brain chemistry dysfunction, or their own over-indulgence in addictive substances and/or activities.

Thus, the war against addiction and the process of healing and rehabilitation is much more a process of "discovery" than of recovery -a process of discovering "normal" —discovering physical health, emotional well-being, and spiritual serenity, developing healthy relationships, a rewarding career, etc. It is the process of discovering a meaningful, rewarding and fulfilling life.

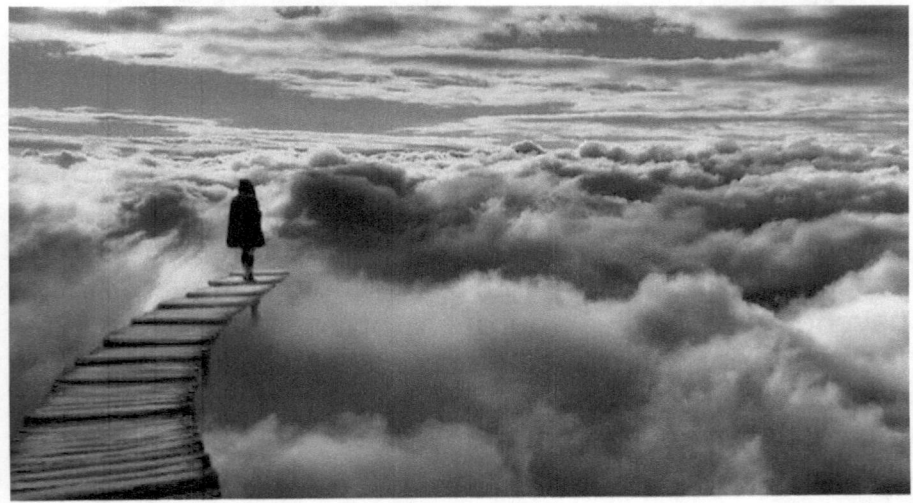

Discovering normal requires a multidisciplinary, multimodal approach to addiction treatment – treatment that involves the addiction sufferer, his or her significant other, the children involved and, when possible, extended family members, friends and co-workers.

The addicted person, their families – and others they are in relationship with – often share a very negative outlook of the future. They have lost their sense of meaning and purpose and have become caught up in what psychologist, Victor Frankl, called "The Mass Neurotic Triad" of depression, addiction and aggression. They share in common the symptoms of this triad – a sense of hopelessness, purposelessness and meaninglessness.

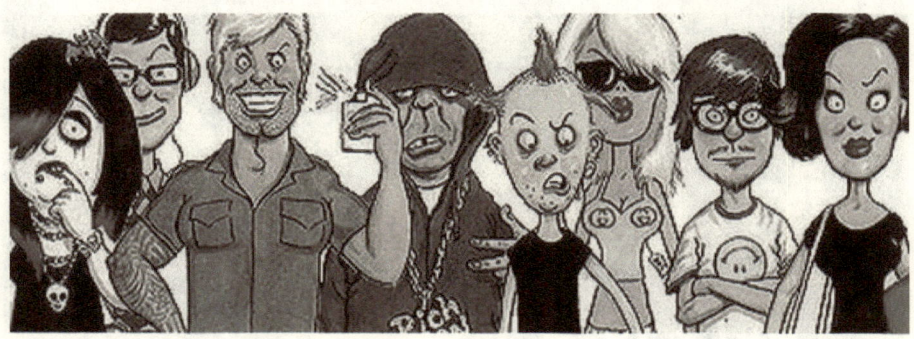

Out of this despair of meaninglessness, there is a growing subculture – a people group seeking to find meaning, purpose and hope outside the norms of society – a society that they feel has let them down and rejected them. It is within this subculture – often referred to as "The Fourth World," that emotional instability, poverty, and violence abounds. It is a world where crime, violence, the abuse of alcohol and illicit substances, aberrant sex and other high-risk activities teem.

These activities are engaged in not so much for pleasure and self-gratification, but rather – research indicates – in an attempt to stimulate the reward pathways within their brain; to anesthetize their inner pain and loss of self-identity; and simply put, to feel "normal."

Attempting to extricate individuals out of this subculture through punishment and/or promised rewards have for the most part failed. It is only within this subculture and through participation in the activities involved therein that the addicted person experiences any sense of normal, or perceived well-being. Successful intervention and lifestyle modification is possible – as treatment has heretofore demonstrated. Utilizing current research and state of the art assessment and treatment techniques, there is more hope now than ever before.

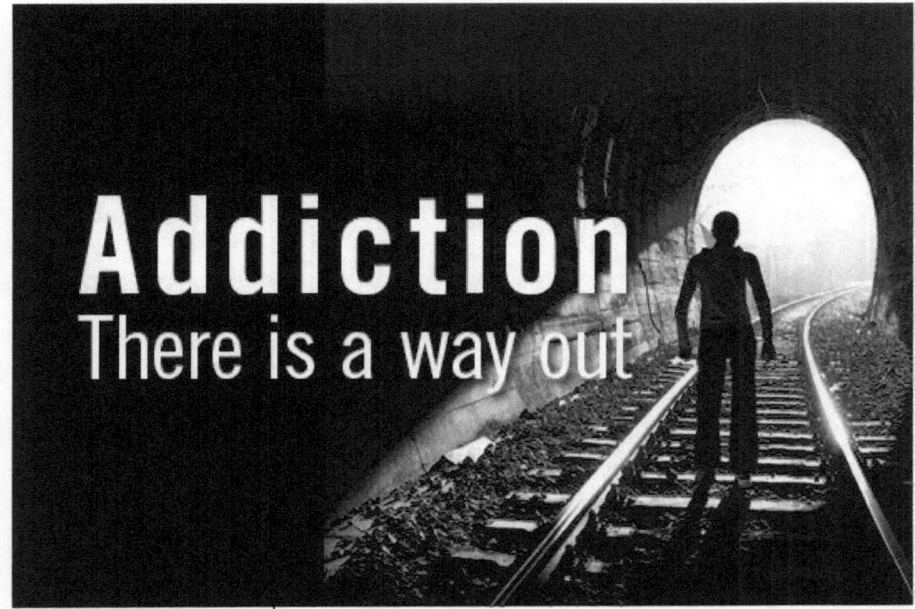

Standing in the light of current and ongoing research, it is time for society to quit criminalizing the addiction sufferer, time for us to give up the concept of legalizing the substances and activities that cause so many so much suffering, and time to medicalize the treatment process. It is high time that we employ medical science to the same degree and in the same fashion that we do when dealing with other diseases.

The "disease concept" of addiction has been around now for several decades, but the acceptance of this concept has been slow among many sectors of the populace outside of the medical and treatment professions. This reticence to accept the disease concept of addiction has, primarily, centered on two arguments:

1.   That while an addiction manifests many disease symptoms, it was self-induced, and

2.   That the locus (or location) of the disease – if it were one – could never be isolated and identified.

These arguments are now moot. Regarding the first argument, many individuals use alcohol and other psychoactive substances without ever becoming addicted while others become addicted almost instantaneously.

The reason? The differences in one's predisposition for addiction —now termed the "Reward Deficiency Syndrome." The second argument has, likewise, been disproved through the discoveries associated with the Reward Deficiency Syndrome. Addiction is a disease (dis-ease), or anomaly, situated within the brain. These anomalies may be genetic, and/or caused by physical injury to the head, by emotional trauma of significant intensity or duration to alter one's brain chemistry, or by one's over indulgence in the substance or activity.

More importantly than the cause, these anomalies within the brain can now be located, measured, diagnosed and treated. Advanced treatment programs are incorporating these current findings and therapeutic modalities, in staffing, program content and intervention modalities.

Key staff members of the treatment team include psychiatrists, psychopathologists, addictionologists, medical assistants, nationally and/or state certified addiction counselors, clergy, pastoral-counselors and other trained assistants. Program content includes components that appropriately address the participant's physical, psychological, spiritual and socio-environmental needs. Collectively they form what has come to be called a Biopsychosociospiritual treatment approach.

Chapter Four
Biopsyshosociospiritual Treatment

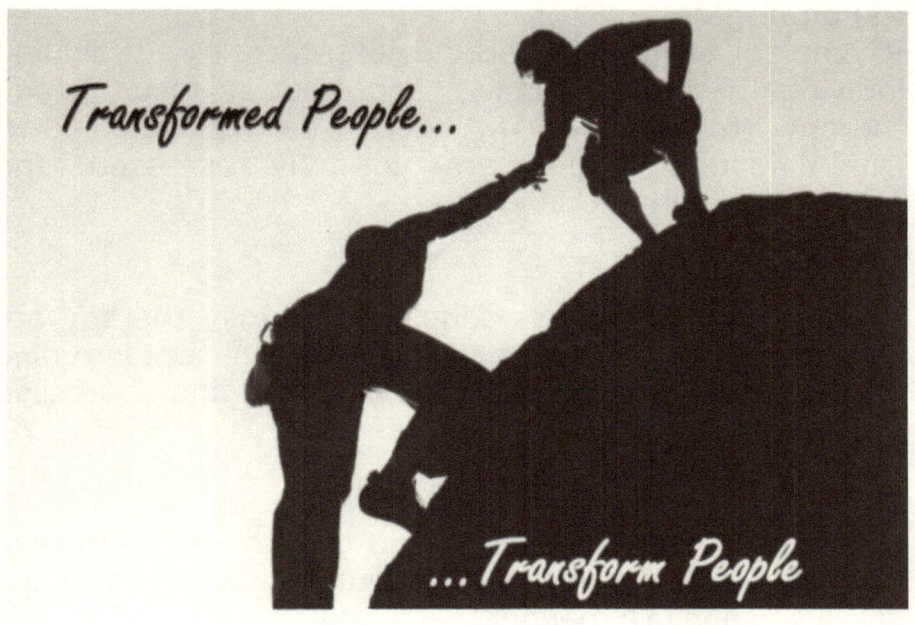

Transformed People...

...Transform People

Biopsychosociospiritual therapy employs specific techniques that address each component:
- Biological or medical
- Psychological
- Sociological
- Spiritual

Biological
Physical needs are addressed through appropriate medical examinations, that ideally include state-of-the art brain-mapping such as the BEAM (Brain Electrical Activity Mapping) or SPECT (Three-dimensional Spectraphotometry).

Treatment episode retention is materially improved through the employment of such methodologies as ariculotherapy (a specialized form of accu-pressure within the ear that stimulates the production of certain hormones), conventional acupuncture and acupressure, nutritional guidance and nutritional supplementation.

Psychological
Psychological needs are addressed by providing individual, couple, family, and special focus group therapy tailored to fit each participant's need. Dual-diagnosis issues are carefully assessed and properly treated.

Sociological
At appropriate intervals couple and family therapy are provided, environmental and sociological factors including job-readiness and job-skills are assessed and addressed therapeutically.

Spiritual
Spirituality, spiritual healing and growth are addressed from an interfaith perspective, outside of the construct of religion and in a manner that is sensitive to participants' varying world views.

While each and every one of these components may demand change to insure a successful therapeutic outcome, the need for such change must be introduced in a manner that appears to meet the goals and objectives of the individual's implicit contract, rather than the explicit plan of the therapeutic team.

Implicit vs. Explicit Treatment Plan
For example, while the explicit plan will no doubt include the goal of achieving and maintaining abstinence from the substances and activities with a high propensity for abuse and addiction, the patient's implicit plan is far more likely to be aimed at preserving or restoring their relationships, avoid incarceration, maintain their employment, etc. While the explicit plan of the therapeutic team must ultimately prevail, the patient must have

some assurance that his/her implicit plan will be met, or it is unlikely that they will remain in treatment.

An effective program incorporates a number of treatment outcomes or goals, objectives and methodologies. They seek to: provide accurate medical and psychological assessments of each participant in sufficient depth to facilitate differentiation between primary and secondary disorders, severity of dependence, co-morbidity of disorders, and personality factors that may affect therapeutic intervention modalities and outcomes.

Treatment Planning

They develop an individualized treatment plan for each client that addresses his or her unique biomedical, psychological, spiritual, and environmental challenges, address the physical well-being of participants incorporating alternative techniques including ariculotherapy, pharmacology, nutratherapy,

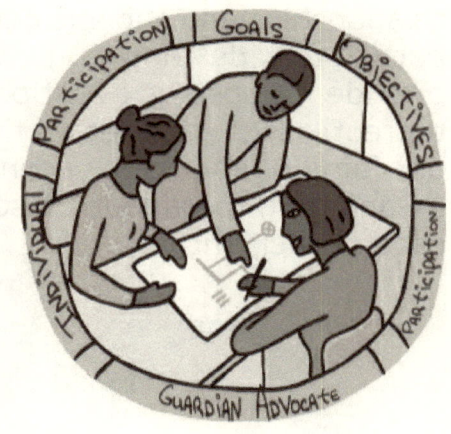

electro-cranial and amino-stimulation of the neurotransmitters.

They help participants gain an accurate understanding of their disease and the rehabilitation or recovery process over the life-span, introduce participants to 12-Step programs and to help them integrate these steps into their plan of recovery and lifestyle of sobriety, encourage each participant in their individual spiritual awakening and unique spiritual walk, meet the educational needs of each participant – making the information imparted as accessible as possible.

They help participants overcome the isolation and fear associated with addictive/compulsive behaviors and achieve positive re-socialization objectives, advocate on behalf of participants, assisting them in the resolution of legal issues including court proceedings, assist each participant in their quest to become a productive member of society and the work force, assist participants and their families in their efforts to resolve relationship issues and make family system adjustments throughout the rehabilitation and recovery process.

They teach participants the necessary relationship and social skills that support healthy interpersonal relationships and support personal recovery, helping each participant develop a personal support system and provide relapse prevention training to the members thereof, assist participants through the adjustment period of family and socioeconomic reentry, develop a meaningful, therapeutic discharge and aftercare plan for each participant.

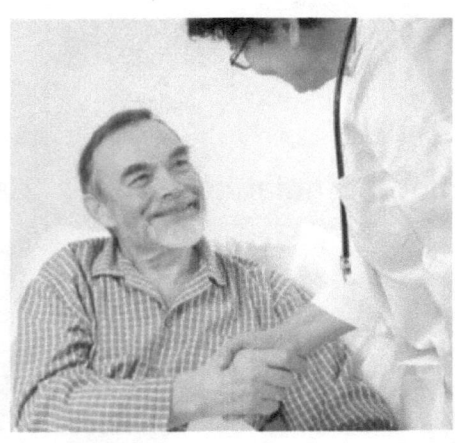

They provide outpatient follow-up services to reinforce the participants' recovery process, network with other service providers in the community, medical personnel, counselors, educators and employers within the community and region to insure that each participant obtains the best therapeutic fit, a complete continuum of care, and understanding.

They network with public regulatory agencies, service providers and private organizations, to insure that participants' varied needs are addressed by the most competent individuals.

The majority of these components are found in most effective programs today, however, more emphasis has been placed on the psychological, spiritual and socio-environmental aspects of treatment than the physical or medical. However, it is the physical problems and effects of the varied addictions that remains the focus of the sufferer.

To these sufferers —those who often prematurely terminate treatment —alternative techniques such as nutritional supplementation, auriculotherapy and/or chiropractic adjustments become important components of effectual treatment. Recent research has demonstrated that attention to the physiological needs of those in treatment increases retention (staying in the program) as well as improving treatment outcomes (results).

One governmental funded research project in Florida demonstrated a 96% retention to clinical discharge when auriculotherapy (a specialized form of acupressure) was incorporated, as compared with a 65.5% retention rate for participants in a similar group without such treatment.

And, in several separate treatment studies, outcomes were significantly improved and recidivism (failure or relapse) rates dramatically reduced by incorporating nutritional supplementation with specific amino acids and vitamin-mineral cofactors to stimulate the production of dopamine, serotonin, norepinephrine, and GABA within the brain's reward pathway (or pain-pleasure center).

The utilization of specific blends of amino acids, vitamins and minerals have been shown to substantially increase treatment outcomes in virtually all those struggling with addictions, those with obsessive-compulsive behaviors (i.e., compulsive gambling and sexual addictions), and those suffering from Attention Deficit Hyperactivity Disorder (ADHD) and Autism.

Researchers in the field of addiction, reporting at the first National Conference on the "Reward Deficiency Syndrome," (RDS) in San Francisco, in November, 2000, state that "as scientists and practitioners, [we] are now convinced that the treatment of RDS associated behaviors should consist of:

•   Physiological and psychological diagnosis (based on genetic testing, brain electro-physiological mapping and psychometric testing);

•   Rebalancing   of the neurotransmitters [within the brain]   (through pharmacological therapies and amino acid based therapy);

•   Neurotransmitter activation (through biofeedback, cranial electrostimulation, acupuncture/auriculotherapy, and   perhaps chiropractic induced subluxation); and

•   Traditional therapies (including psychotherapy, self-help groups, structured aftercare programs, etc.)." [And, spiritual growth.]

The authors were pleased to have the opportunity to attend this conference on behalf of the Professional Associations: the National Association of Forensic Counselors and the National Board of Addiction Examiners Diplomate, and as Executive Director of Alliance Recovery Services, Redding, California.

Conference speakers included:
• Daniel G. Amen, MD, clinical neuroscientist, psychiatrist and medical director of the Amen Clinics, California
• Kenneth Blum, Ph.D., noted author and adjunct professor in neuroscience at the University of North Texas and President of Pharmo-Genomics.
• Michael A. Bozarth, Ph.D., professor of psychology at the State University of New York, noted for his

research in "the neurobiology of the reinforcing effects of abused drugs."

- Eric R. Braverman, MD, pioneer in brain research at Harvard Medical School, founder and director of Path Medical Foundation, and the Brain electrical Activity Mapping (BEAM) diagnostic tool.
- David Comings, MD, Geneticist and Director of the Tourett Syndrome Clinic at the City of Hope National Medical Center.
- Shirley Y. Hill, Ph.D., professor of psychiatry, psychology and human genetics at the University of Pittsburgh.
- Jay M. Holder, DC, C.Ad, DACACD, president and cofounder of the American College of Addictionology and Compulsive Disorders, and developer of the auricuoltherapy techniques previously described.
- Ernest P. Noble, Ph.D., MD, educator, biochemist and clinical psychiatrist, considered by many to be one of the world's foremost leaders in the field of alcohol research.
- David Smith, MD, founder of the Haight-Ashbury Medical Clinics in San Francisco, California during the early drug-explosion of the 60's.
- George Uhl, MD, research scientist with the neuromolecular branch, National Institute on Drug Abuse (NIDA).
- Nora D. Volkow, MD, associate director for Life Sciences at Brookhaven National Laboratory. Dr.. Volkow's work has focused on the neurochemical mechanisms of addiction. She advised the conference on a forthcoming vaccine for cocaine addiction!

While at the conference, we met with some of the cutting-edge scientists and therapists in the field including several we have worked with off and on over the previous two decades. For nearly two decades prior to this conference, we had incorporated nutritional supplementation in the treatment of addicted populations and seen positive results. But, choosing the right supplements was sometimes a guess, at best. Now, however, the technology is available to accurately assess the problem and help practitioners optimize their treatment endeavors.

A Team approach is most helpful in implementing this technology. Select members should be familiar with standard and alternative therapies, and receive training and certification in auricuoltherpy techniques and nutritional therapy. This will take much of the guesswork out of treatment planning and insure some of the highest treatment outcomes available in the addiction treatment field.

Key personnel of a Substance Abuse Program, treating Reward Deficiency Syndrome would be well to include the following disciplines:
- Certified Clinical Psychopathologist,
- Doctoral Addictions Counselor,
- Domestic Violence Counselor
- Certified Clinical Hypnotherapist.
- Medical Doctor,
- Certified Addictionologist
- Licensed Chiropractor.
- Certified Pastoral-Counselor
- Ordained Clergy
- Consultants in Psychiatry, Neurology, Internal Medicine, and Forensic Medicine.

In our next chapter are synopses of several cutting-edge therapy techniques presented at the conference.

Chapter Five
Cutting-edge Techniques

Dr. Kenneth Blum, in his book, *Alcohol and the Addictive Brain,* and in a more recently published article entitled, *Reward Deficiency Syndrome,* that appeared in the American Scientist, 1996, claims to have identified a candidate for genetic manipulation.

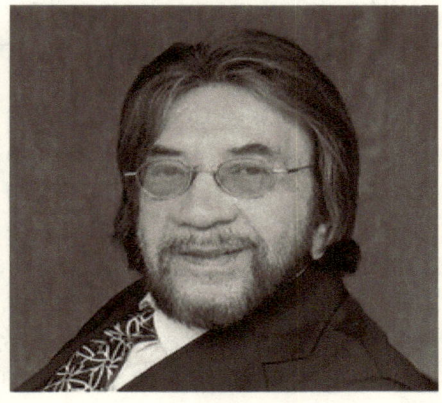

Originally named the alchogene', now called the D2R2 allele (it is a mutation of a normal gene) that is found in up to eighty percent (80%) of alcoholics, drug addicts, compulsive eaters, and pathological gamblers. Carter suggests that *"If they are right, a bit of prudent engineering on a single bit of the human genome could save immeasurable suffering, disease, and premature death"* (Carter, *Mapping The Brain,* pg. 64).

Nutritional Therapy

The ancient Greek Physician, Hippocrates, claimed that *"man is what he eats."* Nutritional Therapy is an approach to healing founded on the belief that food – as God intended –provides the medicine required to achieve and maintain a state of quality health; and that while certain health problems require supplementation beyond that found in a normal, healthy diet, most can be treated with natural, and naturally derived, products instead of pharmacological medicines.

Proponents point out that nutritional therapy is safe for all age groups and sufferers of virtually every physical ailment. Nutritional Therapy is a holistic life-management discipline, as compared to the generally debilitating fad diets that abound.

It involves learning about one's own self, to discover what contributes to one's personal peak in energy, vitality and overall health maintenance. As one nutritional writer has declared, "[natural] food is the cornerstone [made without human hands] which, in our modern life, has been rejected by the builder."

Our modern-day lifestyle seems to be based on speed and instant gratification. We either skip, or hurry through, breakfast; dash out the door –a bit behind schedule –and speed to work, hoping not to get caught violating the law, which escalates our blood pressure. Arriving at work, we immediately get caught up in the pressure of deadlines and performance –working right through our lunch time in an effort to keep caught up.

We work overtime to pay for the numerous "timesaving" appliances we own. We and finally leave work late to dash home, hoping to have enough time for supper with the kids before our evening appointments. The pressure of this lifestyle impels us into eating at fast-food restaurants and "preparing" microwave ready meals –a lifestyle in which "time is of the essence," and the quality of life — including our food –has become secondary.

Eating fast foods on the run, fueling our bodies with short-chain carbohydrates (junk-food) to keep going and sustain the pressure we're under, denies us the privilege, purpose, and the experience of our acquiring, preparing,

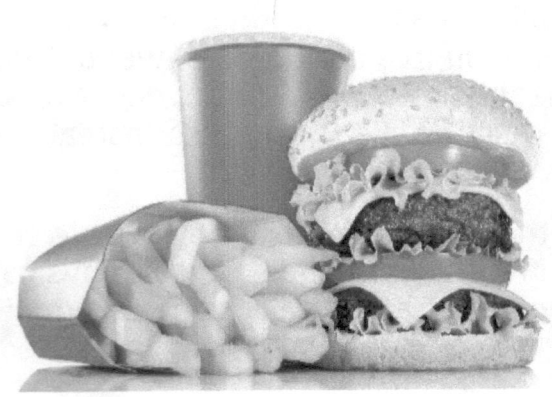 and enjoying our food. Alas, for all the benefits available to man –including our vast agribusiness and neighborhood supermarkets —our food nowadays has less nutritional value than ever before.

The extensive use of chemicals to increase productivity and shorten growing times, the consolidation of the small gardens into huge truck-gardens and hydrophonic farms, and the vast distances agricultural products must be transported to market, has resulted in one of two things:

a)   the produce being harvested before it is truly ripe, or

b)   an increase of processed foods to avoid the waste and spoilage encountered when harvesting at maturity and transporting to market.

Our lifestyle and nutritional patterns are inextricably interwoven, both deriving in part from the familial and cultural traditions one is exposed to, and in part from one's attitude regarding their individual importance to the quality of life. While most of us have little control over the environment that we were raised in, we have almost complete control over our attitude about food and the choices we make. However, to make appropriate food choices, we need accurate information and a correct understanding of a food's impact on our well-being.

Nutritional therapy is based on the belief that every illness has a nutritional basis, the body responding to a deficiency or overabundance of particular nutrients through the manifestation of a disease or group of disease symptoms. In support of this theory, proponents point out that when these nutrients are balanced and appropriate lifestyle changes are made to maintain this balance, the symptoms mitigate or disappear. Thus, most illness is preventable, and most disease curable through proper nutrition.

Proper nutritional therapy is particularly useful in the treatment of hard to diagnose health problems and the so-called incurable diseases such as heart disease, diabetes, arthritis, addictions and eating disorders.

Proper nutrition also mitigates the side effects of chemotherapy, radiation therapy and many drugs. Nutritional therapists point out that while proper nutrition will prevent most illness, nutritional supplementation with vitamins, minerals, herbs and amino acids, is necessary in the treatment of many illnesses.

Critical to proper nutritional supplementation, however, is an understanding that such supplements are themselves a form of medicine —alternative medicines -- which must be administered prudently, with knowledge and wisdom. Herbs are the "raw material" for many pharmaceuticals and are, therefore, of medicinal value in and of themselves.

Amino Acid Therapy

Amino acids form the basic building blocks of life. All of the nearly 40,000 uniquely different proteins within the human body are synthesized from only twenty photogenic amino acids. When our amino acids are in balance, our neurotransmitters are in balance and our neurochemical and electromagnetic equilibrium is achieved, contributing to a sense of happiness, well-being and serenity.

When the amino acids are out of balance, our neurotransmitters are out of balance and our entire neurochemical and electromagnetic equilibrium is disrupted, resulting is the manifestation of disease symptoms such as: anxiety, depression, cognitive processing difficulties, concentration and mental focus difficulties, labile, erratic mood swings, extreme anger, urges, cravings, etc.

While the subject of nutritional deficiencies and nutritional supplementation is far too broad to cover in depth in this text, there are a number of specifics in the field that relate to the treatment of addicts and offenders worthwhile mentioning.

First and foremost, is the fact that nearly all addicts and offenders have a depleted level of Serotonin – which is considered the great civilizing hormone.

Symptoms of Serotonin deficiency include: agitation, anger, rage, anxiety, depression, panic, irritability, low energy level with apathy, self-mutilating behavior, insomnia and/or fitful sleep. In one study involving individuals convicted of domestic violence, eighty-five percent (85%) were found to have deficient levels of Serotinin. And, the deficiency of Serotonin is one of the antecedents to alcoholism since when alcohol is metabolized in the liver, it produces acetaldehyde (a chemical cousin of formaldehyde) which the brain utilizes as a false Serotonin. The inherent problem being that acetaldehyde destroys Serotonin, exacerbating the Problem.

Tryptophan —one of the body's essential amino acids is the precursor, or building material for Serotonin. When ingested in nutrient form, Tryptophan is converted into 5-hydroxy-tryptophan by Tryptophan hydroxylase, which is in turn converted into Serotonin. Tryptophan, in a concentrated form, was outlawed by the Food and Drug Administration during the early 1990's, however, 5-hydroxy-tryptophan —marketed as 5-HTP – is readily available. And recently, pursuant to ongoing research, Tryptophan is one more available.

Another amino acid imbalance commonly found among addicts and offenders is that of Tyrosine the precursor to Dopamine. Tyrosine is not one of the essential amino acids, but is derived from one of the essentials – Phenylalanine. Administered in therapeutic doses, Tyrosine enhances the body's production of Dopa, Dopamine, Norepinepherine and Epinepherine, which are hormones that contribute to the function of the brain's reward pathway, thereby contributing to a sense of pleasure and well-being.

Deficiencies of these hormones contribute to several disorders including Parkinson Disease, Tourette Syndrome, Anhedonia, Restless Leg Syndrome and agitation. All of these disorders respond favorably to the administration of Tyrosine.

Many addicts and offenders report an unusually high level of anxiety —anxiety that triggers many addicts to self medicate with alcohol and marijuana just to feel 'normal.' Anxiety also contributes to the abuse and addiction of a number of pharmaceuticals within the benzodiazipam category. Each of these has significant, harmful side effects that can be avoided by the proper use of a harmless, readily available nutritional supplement — GABA. GABA is a form of endogenous benzodiazipam manufactured within the enteric brain.

Mega-doses of specific vitamins, minerals and amino acids have been found to be as effective as pharmaceuticals in managing drug detoxification and recovery maintenance, treating inchoate anger and rage, anhedonia, anxiety and depression, paranoia and a host of other ills commonly manifest among addicts and offenders.

For example: mega-doses of Vitamin C (as much as 50 grams a day) has been found to be as effective as Methadone in opiate withdrawal –and much safer. The amino acid, Glutamine, effectively curbs the craving for alcohol and high carbohydrate (junk) foods. Niacin and Niacinamide produce a gently sedating effect that is beneficial in the treatment of a wide variety of emotional and neurological disorders including: anxiety, depression, attention deficit disorder, alcoholism, drug addiction, and schizophrenia.

These are just a few of the many benefits of nutritional therapy and its relationship to the field of counseling.

Addiction and offender counselors who desire to offer a holistic approach need to avail themselves of specialized training in nutrition and nutritional therapy, and develop working relationships with professional colleagues who specialize in this area.

To fully comprehend this mind-body-spirit connection and the application of spiritual disciplines, it is essential to understand that addicts and offenders categorically have a sense of inner emptiness within that they seek to compensate for through their obsessive-compulsive behavior patterns. The drivenness in their behavior is really about the fractured, or lost, self and the wounded individual's frantic effort to restore his or her selfhood through the misguided and fruitless "engorging" of an external pacifier, and an external manifestation of being "the greatest" or, as some describe it, "ten feet tall."

The focus of the addictive lifestyle (whether an ingestive addiction such as alcohol, drugs or food; or an activity addiction such as gambling, sex, work, buying, thievery, etc.) is immaterial. It is really an attempt to create an "intimate" relationship with an inanimate object, while at the same time avoiding the pain of self-disclosure that would expose one's shame to a significant other person.

Thus, we create our 'relationships' with things and activities rather than with other people. The alcoholic with his booze, the workaholic with his job, the television junkie with her soaps, the rageaholic with his or her rage, and the criminal with his own superego. Each of them is having a "love affair." Each love affair is a mood-altering experience through which one seeks to avoid the loneliness and pain crying out from his or her shame-bound spirit -- that deep, visceral pain that continually cries for satiation.

Unfortunately, because of the loss of his or her inner self, the addicted individual or codependent is usually unaware of the origin of their pain, but keenly aware of the need to alter his or her mood to temporarily feel better in the very core of his or her being (the "spirit," "chi," "inner- man," etc.). Little do they stop to realize that ingestive addictions, which stimulate their stomach; and the central nervous system stimulants and activities, which stimulate their adrenals, are, in reality, making them feel good temporarily, in almost the right place!

The Enteric or Belly-Brain

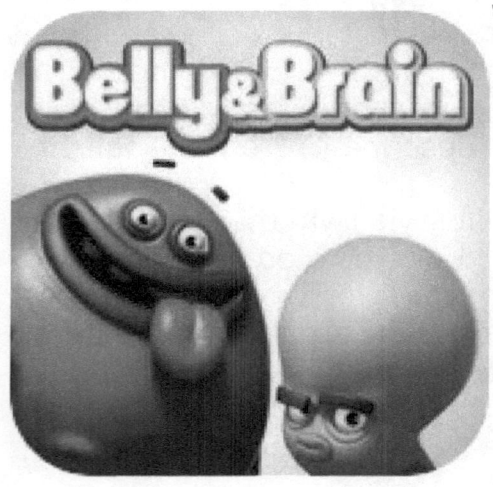

Where is that right place? That "right place" is ... **THE BELLY BRAIN!** Scientists have discovered – or in truth rediscovered - that mankind has a second, and far more sensitive, brain in his inner-being – his stomach, upper intestine and gall bladder.

This second brain, first documented by a 19th century German Neurologist, Leopold Auerbach, was more recently rediscovered by Michael Gershorn, at the University of Columbia in New York.

Once dismissed as just a collection of relay neurons, this "belly-brain" is now recognized as a complex, integrative brain in its own right that is structurally, chemically and operationally specific. It contains approximately 100 billion nerve cells –more than the number of neurons in the spinal cord or frontal cortex. It has both sensory and motor nerves, as well as information processing circuitry.

And, this second brain seems to have a special function. It is connected to our anterior brain through a complex system of neural pathways. But, the two brains –the anterior (in the head) and the enteric (or belly-brain) do not share equal communication functions. The belly-brain selectively sends about nine messages to the anterior brain for every one that it receives back from it!

Furthermore, the belly brain produces and uses a vast array of the so-called "pleasure" or mood-controlling neurotransmitters including: Dopamine, Serotonin, Acetylcholine, GABA, Nitric Oxide and Norepinephrine. Over ninety-five percent (95%) of the body's Serotonin (referred to as the great civilizing neurotransmitter) is created in the gastrointestinal neurons.

The Belly-brain even also creates the greatest amount of natural Benzodiazepines, chemicals of the psychoactive drug group including Xanax and Valium.

The presence of this belly-brain, or Enteric Nervous System was apparently understood –at least in part –by ancient Judaean and Sumerian authors who stated that the spirit of man dwells in his belly or bowels (Proverbs 20:27).

By Divine design, it is from one's spirit, or belly-brain, that one's anterior brain –or mainframe computer –was designed to receive direction and exercise primary control.

Imagine the effect on your life – your self-control – when you artificially stimulate or numb, through alcohol, drugs, sex, codependent relationships, or some other compulsive behavior the reward hormones and neurotransmitters within the belly-brain. Imagine for a moment the confused neuronal messages being sent from your belly-brain to your anterior brain in such circumstance; then you will begin to comprehend the bewildering patterns of aberrant behavior that result.

Moreover, the "fix" achieved through one's compulsive/addictive behavior is only temporary. As it wears off the unresolved, inner pain again calls for the need to mood alter. Each time we yield to the desire to seek a mood-altering fix – with each episode of addictive acting-out —there are more life-damaging consequences which serve to increase one's shame, exacerbating the deep inner pain and fueling the next episode of addictive acting-out.

Then, in an attempt to avoid or limit the life-damaging consequences of acting-out, the addict or codependent begins to focus on the issue of control, seeking the power to control or overcome his or her destructive behavior or addiction. But, the harder he or she seeks to attain control — the more intense one's effort — the more one struggles against his or her own complex nervous system, thereby defeating the belly brain's effort to direct the very control sought after.

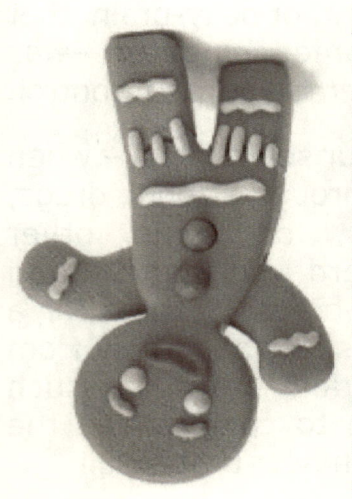

And, the more one concentrates his or her neuronal energy within the anterior (or head) brain, the greater sense of emptiness and pain one experiences within their spirit (gut or belly brain). Lastly, it is the severity, or magnitude of this emptiness or pain, multiplied by the length of time endured that one interprets as the loss of self-identity and self-worth —or shame.

Thus, one lives his life much like the adjacent little gingerbread man —upside down! Rather than being influenced by God, or The Creator, as we understand Him, we live our lives being controlled by those people, places, things and situations around us that we have created love affairs with. When our "best efforts" fail we finally take time to check out our "gut-feeling" (belly-brain or spirit) seeking answers beyond our own reasoning.

The result of living our lives in this manner is that we make ourselves subject to the people, places and things around us. Our focus is external. We come to believe that our state of being at any given moment is being controlled by what happens *to* us rather than what is happening *in* us.

We manipulate this sensory information to the best of our ability through our thoughts and emotions and, only when we are at a total loss, do we then seek answers beyond ourselves —employing the power of the Enteric or belly-brain (or spirit) to transcend our limits. We feel lost —we feel shame (the sense of being less than), so we reach out beyond us. However, operating at that moment in exactly opposite manner of our design, and without guidance, we seek out the very things that produce our addictions.

Then, having once indulged ourselves we feel shame for our inability to control the desire - giving in to the urge to partake. Only when we get our life turned right-side-up again —allowing ourselves, in our spirit, or belly brain, to receive direction from The Unseen, then sending this directive to the anterior brain to determine how to carry it out —do we begin to change, to feel fulfilled and satisfied.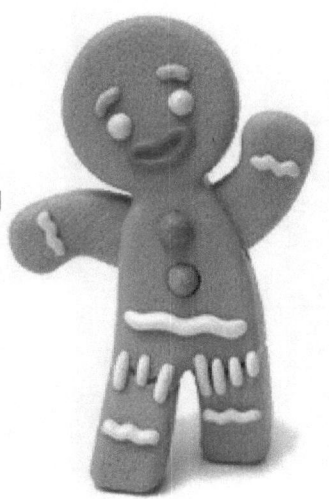

describe the abuse of alcohol and drugs. The Judeo-Christian Bible, more widely known in the Western world, also has a great deal to say on the subjects of crime and addictions.

For example: Genesis records the fact of sibling rivalry culminating in murder within the first household on earth. King Solomon - writing during the tenth century B.C. – advised us that, *"Wine is a mocker and beer a brawler; whoever is led astray by them is not wise"* (Proverbs 20:). Solomon then goes on to tell us the outcome of one who allows himself to be thus led astray:

He asks, *"Who has woe? Who has sorrow? Who has bruises without cause? Who has bloodshot eyes?"* The answer he provides, reveals the chain of addiction. *"Those who linger over wine, those who go in to sample bowls of mixed drink. Do not,"* he warns, *"gaze at wine when it is red, when it sparkles in the cup; when it goes down smoothly! In the end it bites like a snake and poisons like a viper. Your eyes will see strange sights and your mind imagine strange things. You will be like one sleeping on the high seas, in the top of the rigging"* (Pro 23:29-34).

Chapter Six
The Biological Connection

Science and medicine have known for decades that morphological characteristics, character traits, auto immune disorders, certain other diseases, and various physiological traits are transmuted from generation to generation. Similarly, we have more than ample scientific, medical and empirical 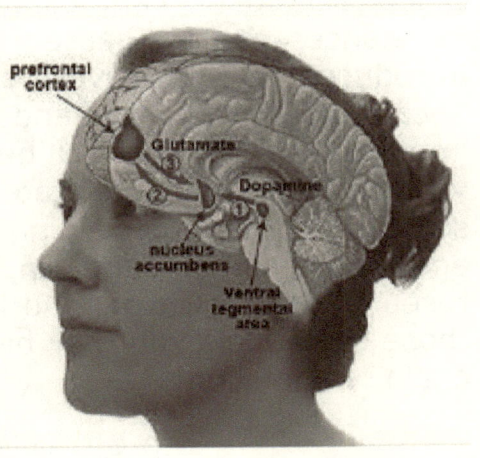 data to prove that mental and emotional strengths and weaknesses, as well as personality disorders can be passed on genetically. Now there is growing evidence to suggest that even behavioral patterns are transgenerationally transmitted.

A growing body of research has established, beyond any reasonable doubt, that behavior alters one's brain chemistry and the genetic mutations thus created become predispositions to these same behavioral patterns that are passed along to the next generation.

It is also now generally accepted that certain brain chemistry imbalances are directly connected to specific resulting behavioral patterns. For example. From these studies, we know that individuals who display a great deal of anger and depression, who act out in patterns of aggression, abuse and violence, generally have an imbalance in one or more of the following brain chemicals: serotonin, dopamine, GABA and endoephenephrine.

This knowledge has also been confirmed through extensive empirical experimentation by psychiatrists who have successfully altered certain behavioral patterns through psychotropic medication.

Since scientists can confirm that these chemical imbalances can be passed on genetically, as well as introduced through severe childhood trauma, a glance back at your family tree and early childhood may reveal important secrets that will help you understand some of your problems and accelerate your healing. The following scientific evidence pertaining to chemical imbalance may add additional guidance in, and impetus for, you to research your own genetic history, as well as that of those individuals you may be seeking to help break the chain of addiction:

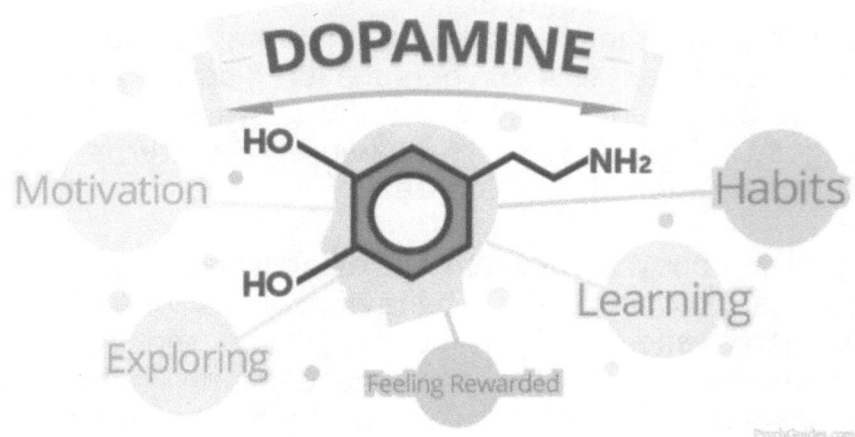

DOPAMINE IMBALANCE: Dopamine is a hormone that regulates motor activity. There are a number of known diseases directly linked to dopamine abnormalities:

1.   Schizophrenia (symptoms include bizarre thoughts, hearing voices, and paranoid behavior).

2.	Parkinson's disease (symptoms include trembling, unbalanced posture, a shuffling walk).

3.	Huntington's chorea (symptoms usually appear after the age of thirty-five and include random twitching and clumsiness, as well as deterioration of mental abilities).

4.	Tourette's syndrome (symptoms include bizarre facial ties, bark-like sounds, and, in about half the cases, uncontrolled cursing).

5.	Attention deficit disorder (symptoms appear early in life and include inattentiveness, impulsive behavior, and sometimes hyperactivity).

6.	Paranoia and paranoid delusions

All of these dopamine-related problems involve some sort of physical or motor dysfunction, although each one also has other unique behavioral symptoms.

Dopamine is a neurotransmitter linked to motor/movement disorders, ADHD, addictions, paranoia, and schizophrenia. Dopamine strongly influences both motor and thinking areas of the brain. One type of Dopamine works in the brain movement and motor system. As this level if dopamine decreases below the "normal range" we begin to experience more motor and gross-movement problems.

Very low levels of Dopamine in the motor areas of the brain are known to produce Parkinson's Disease with symptoms that include:

Muscle rigidity and stiffness

Stooped/unstable posture

Loss of balance and coordination

Gait (walking pattern) disturbance

Slow movements and difficulty with voluntary movements

Small-step gait/walking

Aches in muscles

Tremors and shaking

Fixed, mask-like facial expression

Slow, monotone speech

Impairment of fine-motor skills

Falling when walking

Impairment in cognitive/intellectual ability

Dopamine in the thinking areas of the brain might be considered the neurotransmitter of focus and attending. Lower than normal levels impair one's ability to focus on their environment or to "lock on" to tasks, activities, or conversations. This level of Dopamine deficiency makes concentration and focus very difficult. Low levels of Dopamine are also associated with Attention-Deficit Hyperactivity Disorder (ADHD).

At the other end of the Dopamine balance, as Dopamine levels in the brain begin to rise, we become excited and energized. But, when Dopamine levels become excessive, we tend to become suspicious and paranoid. Finally, we become hyper-stimulated by our environment. With low levels of Dopamine, we can't focus while with abnormally high levels of Dopamine our focus becomes narrowed and so intense that we are inclined to focus on everything in our environment as though it were directly related to our personal experience and well-being.

Mildly low elevations in Dopamine are associated with addictions. Nicotine, cocaine, and other substances produce a feeling of excited euphoria by artificially increasing Dopamine levels in the brain. Too much of these chemicals/substances and we feel "wired." Just like increased levels of Dopamine make us hyper-stimulated, we begin paying too much attention to our environment due to being over-stimulated and unable to separate what's important and what is not.

In an ADHD child, low levels of Dopamine don't allow the child to focus or attend to anything in the environment. The child is physically hyperactive when running about the room or switching from activity-to-activity due to their lack of focus. As Dopamine levels increase above the normal range, our ability to focus increases to the point of our becoming paranoid.

Moderately high Dopamine levels make us defensive, feeling on-guard, suspicious, and prone to misinterpret experiences in the environment. This state is known as an "idea of reference" in psychiatry. In this state, we begin thinking that unrelated experiences are suddenly directly related to us. People observed talking across the street are now believed to be talking about us. As Dopamine increases further, it can become so intense that we believe the radio, television, and newspaper contain secret messages directed to us, or about us.

It's as though we are attempting to incorporate/add everything we witness into our life-experience. Planes flying overhead are, we think, snapping pictures of us and motorists talking on cellular phones are calling in to make a report against us. Our speed of thought increases and races wildly in an attempt to keep up with and add all we see into our environment.

In an attempt to make sense of it all, we may become extremely religious, paranoid, or grandiose, feeling like we are a very important, special person. Increased Dopamine also increases the perception of our senses, much like turning up the volume in all our senses – hearing, vision, taste, smell, and touch.

As Dopamine levels increase, the noises we heard over-loudly suddenly become auditory hallucinations. Our inner thoughts are now being heard outside of our body. These "voices" begin talking to us and are known to take different forms such as derogatory put-downs, religious directives, commands (telling us to do this or that), or they may be sexually motivating.

If Dopamine levels stay high, hallucinations (experiencing something that is not truly there in reality) will soon develop in all our senses. We may begin seeing faces in clouds, carpets, or patterns. We may sense the touch of spirits or movements inside our body. We may experience unusual smells or tastes.

Heightened levels of Dopamine in the brain can even cause us to lose our contact with reality. We begin to experience life as though we were living in a science-fiction movie. We begin to develop unusual, often bizarre ideas about what is happening to us. With our paranoia, we may experience delusions (false beliefs) of persecution or may think we have super powers (delusions of grandiosity). We may believe we can predict the future or read other's minds.

These high levels of Dopamine are found in Schizophrenia, drug intoxication, and other psychotic conditions where the ability to distinguish the inner world from the outer, or real, world is impaired.

Dopamine levels typically change very slowly. Patients who develop Paranoia and/or Schizophrenia often experience a gradual increase in Dopamine levels over several years - also experiencing an increase in the severity of symptoms over those years.

A typical high school or college student may develop a sense of being on-edge or experience unusual feelings, gradually becoming suspicious and feeling alienated, moving gradually into auditory hallucinations, and finally developing bizarre false beliefs (delusions) of persecution or exaggerated self-importance over the next several years. Stress can often rapidly increase Dopamine, but it still rarely happens overnight.

When an individual becomes psychotic, paranoid, and hallucinates in only a few days, one should strongly suspect medication/drug intoxication or a neurological event – something that could increase Dopamine levels dramatically and almost instantly. The prolonged use of amphetamines/methamphetamines (speed) or steroids can produce a loss of reality and sudden paranoia.

When this occurs, a construction worker taking methamphetamine, or "street speed" to increase his work productivity may believe that his hand or foot is talking to him (auditory hallucinations) and decide to cut it off. The sudden presence of psychosis (hallucinations, delusions, paranoia, etc.) in an individual with a history of prior normal adjustment would suggest the need for intensive medical and neurological work-up.

SEROTONIN IMBALANCE:
Serotonin is called the "great inhibitor" or the "civilizing" brain chemical. Some researchers believe excessively low Serotonin levels may contribute to the following:

Serotonin

1.   Aggressive behavior

2.   Alcohol abuse and dependency

3.   Arson

4.   Borderline personality disorder (long-term unstable behavior)

5. Bulimia

6. Migraine headaches

7. Premenstrual tension (PMS)

8. Violent behavior

9. Violent suicide or homicide

10. Clinical depression

On the other hand, excessively high seretonin levels may contribute to things such as:

1. Autism (symptoms generally appear within the first year of life; child begins to with draw from all human relationships and usually does not respond to human affection)

2. Infantile spasms

3. Bipolar, Manic-depressive Personality Disorder

4. Schizophrenia

5. Some forms of Mental Retardation

When Serotonin receptors are hypersensitive, this may result in:

1. Obsessive-compulsive Personality Disorder

2. Severe Anxiety and Panic attacks

Serotonin, first isolated in 1933, is the neurotransmitter that has been identified as the culprit in multiple psychiatric disorders including depression, obsessive-compulsive disorder, anorexia, bulimia, body dysmorphic disorder (i.e., a nose that doesn't look 'perfect' to the individual, even after having numerous surgeries), social anxiety, various phobias, etc.

Serotonin is a major mood regulator and is involved in numerous bodily processes such as sleep, libido, body temperature, auto-immune functions, etc.

A good way to understand the function of Serotonin is to employ the metaphor of an automobile. Most vehicles in the United States are made to cruise at about seventy miles an hour. This is perfect for driving on the interstate highways when taking your summer vacation or traveling to visit relatives. However, if you were to drive that same automobile on a racetrack day-after-day, at say one hundred thirty miles an hour, the engine would run much hotter than normal, the motor oil would burnout or evaporate, and components of the engine and running gear would begin to fail. Serotonin is – in a sense – the motor oil of the brain.

Much like our normal stock automobile, built for highway driving, that would begin to fail if used on a racetrack, our bodily systems will begin to fail is subjected to a high stress lifestyle for a prolonged period of time. This occurs because under stress we use more Serotonin than our body can replace during the same time period.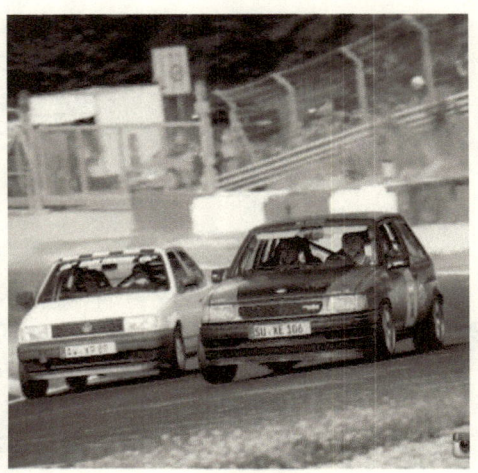

Envision for a moment the pressures that you are under: your responsibilities, the difficulties you are presently facing, environmental issues such as poor housing, living in a rough neighborhood, etc., and sociological problems such as marriage difficulties, parenting problems, troubles with co-workers, etc. prolonged exposure to these stressors gradually depletes one's Serotonin level.

Then, with depleted levels of Serotonin, if we continue to "hang on" to these stressors, we will begin to develop Serotonin deficiency symptoms such as severe stress-related depression.

Referring again to our automobile metaphor; a vehicle can be one, two, perhaps even three quarts low on oil and still operate normally; but if the oil level continues to drop, there comes a point when it becomes critically low. How quickly this happens depends on the load the engine is operating under, i.e., mountain driving is more demanding then cruising through the valley. Add to this a trunk load of stones and a car full of people. Before long, the automobile will cease to function normally, and unless the load is diminished, it will eventually fail.

Our brain function is somewhat like that automobile. While it appears to function normally when our Serotonin is a bit low (say one or two quarts by comparison), our ability to manage stress becomes impaired. This load then depletes our Serotonin even more until we begin to develop sleep disorders, depression and related symptoms.

As our Serotonin level drops lower we begin experiencing concentration and attention problems. We become scatterbrained and poorly organized. Routine tasks begin to seem overwhelming. Our ability to plan our day becomes more difficult resulting in tasks taking longer and longer to complete. Eventually our normal functioning becomes compromised .

At this point we may develop memory problems such as misplacing our car keys. We may also become disorganized and make poor judgments such as putting frozen food in the oven, or odd things in the refrigerator. We may call someone on the phone and then forget who we called, or why we called them. We might go to the grocery store and then wonder what we came for, or tell people the same thing over and over again.

These functionality problems increase our stress, causing our Serotonin level to drop still lower. At this point we may become clinically depressed, even suicidal. Major changes begin occurring in bodily functions that are regulated by Serotonin. We may begin experiencing the following symptoms and manifesting the following behaviors:

Chronic fatigue. Despite sleeping extra hours and naps, we remain tired. There is a sense of being "worn out"

Sleep disturbance, typically we can't go to sleep at night. Our thoughts seem to be racing. "Our mind just won't shut up!"

Early-morning awakening is also common, typically around 4:00 am, at which point going back to sleep is difficult, since our thoughts begin racing once more.

Appetite disturbance is present. We either experience a loss of appetite and subsequent weight loss, or a craving for sweets and carbohydrates when the brain is trying to make more Serotonin.

Total loss of sexual interest is present. In fact, there is usually a loss of interest in most everything, including those activities and interests that have been enjoyed in the past.

Social withdrawal is common - not answering the phone, rarely leaving our house or apartment, we often stop calling friends and family, and even withdraw from social events.

Emotional sadness and frequent crying spells are common.

Self-esteem, self-confidence and competence are diminished.

Body sensations change. Due to Serotonin's role as a body regulator, we experience hot flushes and temperature changes, headaches, and stomach distress.

Change in personality - a sense that our sense of humor has left and our basic temperament has changed.

We begin to take everything very personally. Comments, glances, and situations are viewed personally and negatively. If someone speaks to you, it irritates you. If they don't speak, you become angry and feel ignored.

Your family may have the sense that you have kind of "faded away." You talk less, smile less, and sit for hours gazing into nothingness, noticing no one.

Your behavior becomes odd. Family members may find you up, sitting in the dark in the kitchen at 4:00 am.

Individuals can live many years with low level or moderate depression called Dysthymia. They develop compensations for the lack of sleep and other symptoms. They begin using sleep medication or alcohol to get some sleep. Being chronically unhappy and pessimistic, they explain their situation with "It's just my life!" They may not fully recognize their own depressive symptoms.

Very low levels of Serotonin typically bring people to the attention of their family physician, their employer, or other sources of help. Severe Serotonin loss produces symptoms that are truly difficult to ignore. Not only are severe symptoms present, but also the brain's ideations, or thinking process becomes very uncomfortable and even torturing. When Serotonin is severely low, you will experience some if not all of the following:

Thinking speed will increase. You may have difficulty controlling your own thoughts. You tend to focus on torturing memories and find it difficult to stop thinking about these uncomfortable memories or images.

You become emotionally numb! You don't know how you feel about your life, marriage, job, family, future, significant other, etc. It's as though all your feelings have been turned off. If asked by others how you feel - your response might be "I don't really know!"

Crying outbursts will surface, suddenly crying with little or no warning.

Behavioral outbursts will also surface. If you break the lead in a pencil, you may throw the pencil across the room. Temper tantrums may surface. You may storm out of offices or public places. You begin getting angry easy and have difficulty controlling its expression.

Escapism fantasies begin. The most common - Hit the Road! The brain will suggest packing up your personal effects and leaving your family and community.

Memory torture will begin. Your brain, thinking at 100 miles an hour or more, will search your memories for your most traumatic or unpleasant experiences. You become preoccupied with horrible experiences that may have happened ten, twenty, or even thirty years ago. You will relive the death of loved ones, divorce, childhood abuse - whatever the brain can find to torture you with. And, you'll feel like it happened yesterday.

You'll have Evil Thoughts. New mothers may have thoughts about smothering their infants. Thoughts of harming or killing others may appear. You may be tortured by dark images/pictures in your memory. It's as though the brain finds your most uncomfortable weak spot, then terrorizes you with it.

Serotonin a major bodily regulator, and when Serotonin is this low your body becomes unregulated. You'll experience changes in body temperature, aches/pains, muscle cramps, bowel/bladder problems, smothering sensations, etc. The "Evil Thoughts" then tell you those symptoms are due to a terminal disease. Depressed folks never just have gas. They believe it's colon cancer. A bruise is leukemia.

You may develop a Need-for-Change Panic. You'll begin thinking that a change in lifestyle (Mid-life Crisis!), a divorce, an extramarital affair, a new job, or a Corvette will change your mood. About 70 percent of career jobs are abandoned at this time as depressed individuals gradually fade away from their life. Most extramarital affairs also occur at this time.

Since depressed Serotonin levels are related to obsessive-compulsive disorders, you may find yourself starting to count things, become preoccupied with germs/disease, excessively worry that appliances are turned off or doors locked, worry that televisions must be turned off on an even-numbered channel, etc. You may develop rituals involving safety and counting, or making lists of meaningless things.

Whatever normal personality traits, quirks, or attitudes you have, will suddenly be increased at least threefold. A perfectionist will suddenly become anxiously overwhelmed by the messiness of their environment or distraught over leaves that fall each minute to land on their recently raked lawn. Penny-pinchers will suddenly become preoccupied with electric and water consumption in their home.

A "triggering event" may produce bizarre behavior. Already moderately low in Serotonin, an animal bite or scratch may make you become suddenly preoccupied with rabies. A media story about the harmful effects of radiation may make you remember a teenage tour you took through the local nuclear power plant, and you suddenly feel that all your symptoms are the result of exposure to radiation.

When you reach the bottom of "severely low" Serotonin, the "garbage truck" will arrive. Everyone with severely low Serotonin is told the same thing. You will be told:

1)   You're a bad spouse, parent, child, employee, etc.,

2)   You are a burden to those who love or depend on you,

3)   You are worsening the lives of those around you,

4)   Those who care about you would be better if you weren't there,

5)   You would be better if you weren't around, and

6)   You, and those around you would be better off if you were totally out of the picture.

7)   At that point, you develop suicidal thoughts.

Clinical Depression is perhaps the most common mental health problem encountered in practice. One in four adults will experience clinical depression within their lifetime. Depression has been called the "common cold" of mental health practice. It is both very common and much easier to treat today than in the past. Treatment for depression, as might be expected, involves increasing levels of Serotonin in the brain.

Like all neurotransmitters, we can also have too much Serotonin. While elevated levels of Serotonin produce a sense of well-being, bliss, and "oneness with the universe," too much Serotonin can produce a life-threatening condition known as Serotonin Syndrome (SS). SS is most likely to occur by accident when an individual who has suffered from depression combines two or more Serotonin-increasing medications or substances.

Serotonin Syndrome (SS) produces violent trembling, profuse sweating, insomnia, nausea, teeth chattering, chilling, shivering, aggressiveness, overconfidence, agitation, and malignant hypothermia. Emergency medical treatment is required, utilizing medications that neutralize or block the action of Serotonin as the treatment for Serotonin Syndrome (SS).

Like Dopamine, Serotonin can be accidentally increased or decreased by the use of psychoactive substances and certain medications. One form of birth control medicine is known to produce severe depression since it lowers Serotonin levels.

A specific medication for acne has also been linked with depression and suicidal ideation. For this reason, it is important to inform your physician if you are taking any medication for depression. Also avoid combining antidepressants with any herbal substances reported to be of help in Depression such as St. John's Wort.

NOREPINEPHRINE IMBALANCE

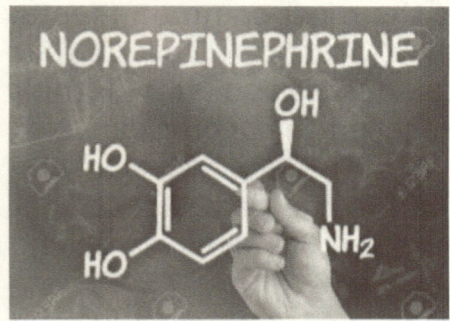

Norepinephrine (NE), an endogenous form of adrenaline made within the human body, is the neurotransmitter often associated with the "fight or flight" response to stress.

Strongly linked to physical responses and reactions, it can increase heart rate and blood pressure as well as create a sense of panic and overwhelming fear and dread. Similar to adrenaline, it sets one's threshold levels to stimulation and arousal.

Emotionality, anxiety and depression are related to norepinephrine levels in the brain, and this neurotransmitter seems to maintain the balance between agitation and depression. Low levels of norepinephrine are associated with a loss of alertness, poor memory, and depression.

Norepinephrine appears to be the neurotransmitter of "arousal" and for that reason, lower-than-normal levels of this neurotransmitter produce below-average levels of arousal and interest, a symptom found in several psychiatric conditions including depression and ADHD. For this reason medications for depression 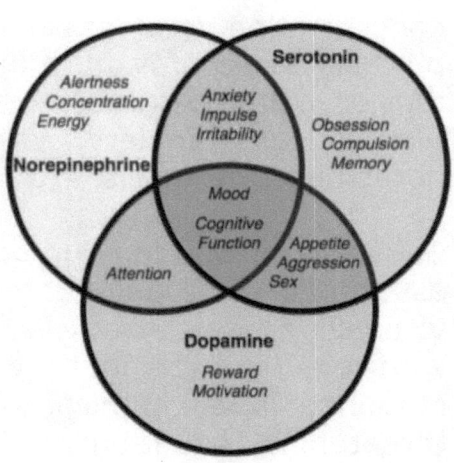 and ADHD often target both dopamine and norepinephrine in an attempt to restore both to normal level.

Mild elevations in our norepinephrine levels produce heightened arousal, something also known to be produced by stimulants. This arousal is considered pleasurable and several "street drugs" such as cocaine and amphetamines work by increasing the brains level of norepinephrine. This increased sense of arousal is pleasurable, linking these substances to their potential for addiction.

Research indicates that some individuals intentionally use antidepressants to develop a state of "hypomania" or emotional elation and physical arousal in this same manner. For that reason, individuals using modern antidepressants are often cautioned to notify their treating physician/psychiatrist if they become "too happy".

Moderately high levels of norepinephrine create a sense of arousal that becomes physically and psychically uncomfortable. Remember, this neurotransmitter is strongly involved in creating physical reactions, moderate increases create worry, anxiety, increased startle reflex, jumpiness, fears of crowds & tight places, impaired concentration, restless sleep, and physical changes. The physical symptoms may include rapid fatigue, muscle tension/cramps, irritability, and a sense of being on edge. Almost all anxiety disorders involve elevated norepinephrine levels.

Severe and sudden increases in norepinephrine are associated with panic attacks. Perhaps the best way to visualize a panic attack is to remember the association with the "flight or fight" response. The "flight or fight" response is a chemical reaction to a dramatic and threatening situation in which the brain produces excessive amounts of norepinephrine and adrenaline. This gives an individual extra strength, increased energy/arousal, muscle tightness (for fighting or running), and a desperate sense that we must do something immediately.

This animal response was no doubt activated in early man when a bear showed up at his cave or when faced with a tiger in the woods. In modern times, imagine your reaction if while calmly watching television, someone or something started trying to knock your front door in to attack you. In the "flight or fight" reaction, your brain and body chemistry prepare you to either run from the situation or fight to the death!

A panic attack is the activation of the "flight or fight" chemical reaction without a bear at the door. It's as though our self-protection response is kicking-off accidentally, when no real life-threatening situation is present. Known now as panic attacks, they can surface at the grocery, at church, or when you least expect it.

As norepinephrine is a fast-acting neurotransmitter, the panic attack may last less than ten minutes (but it feels like hours!). And, when you experience one, you'll be rattled/shaken for several hours thereafter. Panic attacks are strong physical and chemical events and include the following symptoms:

Palpitations, pounding heart or rapid heart rate

Sweating and body temperature changes

Trembling or shaking

Shortness of breath of smothering sensations

Choking sensations

Chest pain and discomfort

Nausea or stomach distress

Dizziness, lightheadedness, or feeling faint

Sense of unreality, as though you are outside yourself

Fear of losing control or going crazy

Fear of dying

Numbness and tingling throughout the body

Chills and hot flushes

Going back to our automobile metaphor, a panic attack is the equivalent of seeing all of your dashboard warning lights coming on and flashing instantaneously and simultaneously. Your stress level is too high. Panic attacks, or surges of norepinephrine, can occur by accident as when created by the use of certain medications or illicit drugs. The medications for certain medical conditions can cause a panic attack or increase our level of anxiety. Medications often used for asthma, for example, can create anxiety or panic attacks. Drugs of abuse are the most common cause.

Treatment for excessively high levels of norepinephrine, as found in anxiety and panic disorders, involves decreasing neurotransmitter levels directly or using medications that increase another neurotransmitter which inhibits or decreases the action of norepinephrine. One of these inhibiting neurotransmitters is GABA, also known as Gamma-Aminobutyric Acid.

GABA IMBALANCE

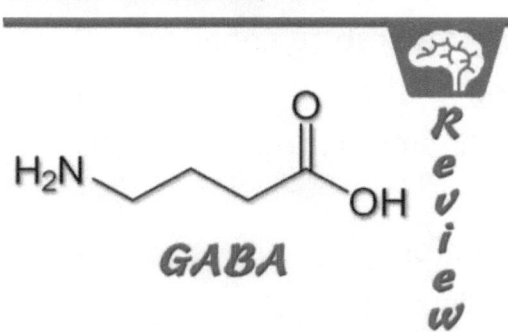

Gamma-Aminobutyric Acid (GABA) is a neurotransmitter that is inhibitory in function. That is, it decreases the ability of other neurotransmitters to work. GABA is involved in our level of excitability. Rather than encouraging communication between cells such as Dopamine, Serotonin or Norepinephrine, GABA reduces, discourages, and blocks this communication. This neurotransmitter is important in brain areas involving emotion and anxiety.

When GABA is in the normal range in the brain, we are not overly aroused or anxious. At the same time, we have appropriate reactions to situations in our environment. Resorting to our metaphor of the automobile, GABA is the governor on the engine, the communication speed controller. It makes certain all brain communications are operating at the right speed and at the correct level of intensity.

Too little GABA in the brain, the communication becomes out of control, over-stimulated, and chemically unstable. Too much GABA and we become overly relaxed and sedated, often to the point that normal reactions are impaired.

Deficient levels of GABA are associated with Bipolar Disorder with Mania. With GABA levels below average, the brain is over-stimulated. We begin talking rapidly, staying up for days at a time, and develop wild and grandiose ideas. When in a Manic state, we are so "high" we are usually out of control.

12 MAIN FACTORS THAT REDUCE GABA LEVELS IN THE BODY

- Too much loud noise
- Lack of glutamine
- Exessive electromagnetic radiations
- Low levels of vitamin B6 and B1
- Lack of minerals such as iron, zinc and manganese
- High amount of caffeine
- Chronic stress
- Alcohol withdrawal
- Chronic pain
- Exposure to lead and mecury
- Not enough sleep
- Low levels of progesterone

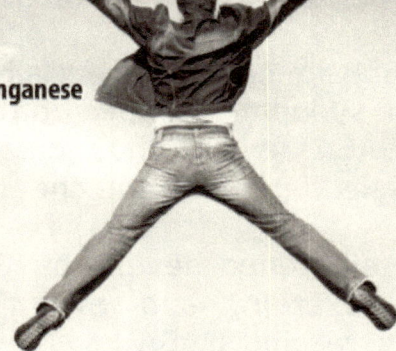

GABA-Supplement.com

Social problems are quick to develop, often due to hyper-sexuality, excessive spending, reckless decisions, risk-taking behavior, and grandiose ideas. We may feel so good that we think we are a heavenly spirit, an intellectual genius, or someone possessing extraordinary powers. I know of one individual who locked himself in his mobile home and spent one week rewriting the New Testament in "hillbilly". Another, with limited education, began purchasing books on the Theory of Relativity by Albert Einstein, sensing he may be able to use the information to invent "warp drive".

Low levels of GABA are also associated with problems of poor impulse control, including clinical conditions such as compulsive gambling, pornography addictions, temper tantrums, and stealing. When GABA is low in the brain, impulsive behaviors are not inhibited (stopped) by logical or reasonable thinking.

Low levels of GABA are also associated with epilepsy or seizure disorders. If we imagine a seizure as a type of electrical storm, the seizure begins at one location in the brain then rushes across and through the brain like a sudden storm. Low levels of GABA make it easy for the brain to develop seizures which is why seizures are part of the withdrawal syndrome for many substances that work with GABA such as alcohol and tranquilizers (benzodiazepams - Xanax, Ativan, Librium, Valium, etc.).

Substances that artificially maintain a high level of GABA, if suddenly stopped, often creates a dramatic drop in GABA levels, thus creating the risk for withdrawal seizures due to the chemical instability that is created.

Heightened levels of GABA produce more control, relaxation, and even sedation. Alcohol works by increasing GABA levels, which is why all body systems are relaxed at first, then sedated to the point when one manifests slurred speech, unsteady gait, and foggy thinking.

Alcohol withdrawal, or the sudden severe drop of high GABA levels, produce a low GABA level and the possibility of seizures. Withdrawal from benzodiazepines is known to follow the same pattern. Taking forty or more milligrams of Valium for two years, and suddenly stopping all medication, will likely produce a seizure.

Medications for anxiety create relaxation and a decrease in anxiety by increasing GABA levels in the brain. Alcoholic beverages work in the same manner; the alcohol increasing GABA levels to produce mild euphoria, loss of social anxiety, and other symptoms of intoxication. Excessive intake of benzodiazepines and/or alcohol is extremely dangerous as the high GABA level actually suppresses the communication between brain neurons - sometimes to the point of a quenching all communication between neurons - also known as death.

Medications for seizures, impulse control problems, and Bipolar Disorder, Mania all work by increasing the GABA levels without creating an accompanying euphoria. Lithium and anti-seizure medications all work by raising GABA into the normal range, thus lowering the possibility of seizures and producing brain chemical stability. As GABA is the neurotransmitter policeman, changes in GABA can influence all neurotransmitters but especially norepinephrine.

Not only do these neurotransmitter imbalances create thought process disorders that impair one's functioning and alters one's behavior, aberrant behavior that artificially disrupts the balance of these chemicals ultimately creates the same physiological and psychological disorders. Thus, substances of abuse,, compulsive activities such as gambling, hyper-sexual activity, and over-stimulation through excitement, deprivation of rest, etc., can mature into these and other disorders.

Even more concerning, is the fact that as these disorders become established, permanent mutations are taking place in our DNA, or genetic makeup that will be passed along to the next generation. For example: When doctors artificially stimulate dopamine, or inhibit serotonin, it often results in increased aggression and sexual activity, affecting the individual's offspring as well as the individual themselves.

These findings further support the biological/behavioral connection. Dopamine is connected to what we commonly call the "pleasure centers" in the brain. It has long been thought that most addictive drugs and compulsive activities prompt a sudden release of dopamine which leads to the theory that addicts are self-medicating imbalances in dopamine levels when taking their drugs.

Studies using rats demonstrate that the desire for pleasure is even more pronounced than that for food. Repeated studies show that rats will choose drugs over food, even to the point of starving themselves to death.

For individuals suffering from addictions, dopamine/serotonin or Norepinephrine/GABA imbalances can present a lethal double whammy. Too little of either one can encourage addiction as the body desperately tries to adjust these levels. Add to this the emotional and environmental pain that triggers self-medication, and it is easy to understand why addiction is such an overwhelming societal problem.

It is a pattern of self-destruction that should not be taken lightly if you discover it lurking in your family tree. For additional information see the book, *"Growing Beyond Our Genetics: Adolescence & Beyond, Potter, J.V. & P.M., Advocare Publishing Co., Anderson, California, 2007.*

Chapter Seven
The Addiction Gene

THE RECOVERY EMPORIUM
Reward Deficiency Syndrome - Article, The Reward Deficiency Syndrome, The American Scientist,' by Kenneth Blum, John G. Cull, Eric R. Braverman & David E. Comings.

"In 1990 one of us published with his colleagues a paper suggesting that a specific genetic anomaly was linked to alcoholism (Blum et al. 1990).

Unfortunately it was often erroneously reported that they had found the "alcoholism gene," implying that there is a one-to-one relation between a gene and a specific behavior. Such misinterpretations are common. Readers may recall accounts of an "obesity gene," or a "personality gene."

Needless to say, there is no such thing as a specific gene for alcoholism, obesity or a particular type of personality. However, it would be naive to assert the opposite, that these aspects of human behavior are not associated with any particular genes. Rather the issue at hand is to understand how certain genes and behavioral traits are connected.

In the past five years we have pursued the association between certain genes and various behavioral disorders. In molecular genetics, an association refers to a statistically significant incidence of a genetic variant (an allele) among genetically unrelated individuals with a particular disease or condition, compared to a control population. In the course of our work we discovered that the genetic anomaly previously found to be associated with alcoholism is also found with increased frequency among people with other addictive, compulsive or impulsive disorders.

The list is long and remarkable - it comprises alcoholism, substance abuse, smoking, compulsive overeating and obesity, attention-deficit disorder, Tourette's syndrome and pathological gambling. We believe that these disorders are linked by a common biological substrate, a "hardwired" system in the brain (consisting of cells and signaling molecules) that provides pleasure in the process of rewarding certain behavior.

Consider how people respond positively to safety, warmth and a full stomach. If these needs are threatened or are not fully met, we experience discomfort and anxiety. An inborn chemical imbalance that alters the intercellular signaling in the brain's reward process is triggered which could supplant an individual's feeling of well being with anxiety, anger or a craving for a substance that can alleviate the negative emotions. This chemical imbalance manifests itself as one or more behavioral disorders for which one of us (Blum) has coined the term "reward deficiency syndrome."

This syndrome involves a form of sensory deprivation of the brain's pleasure mechanisms. It can be manifested in relatively mild or severe forms that follow as a consequence of an individual's biochemical inability to derive reward from ordinary, everyday activities. We believe that we have discovered at least one genetic aberration that leads to an alteration in the reward pathways of the brain. It is a variant form of the gene for the dopamine D2 receptor, called the Al allele. This is the same genetic variant that we previously found to be associated with alcoholism.

In this review we shall look at evidence suggesting that the A1 allele is also associated with a spectrum of impulsive, compulsive and addictive behaviors. The concept of a reward deficiency syndrome unites these disorders and may explain how simple genetic anomalies give rise to complex aberrant behavior.

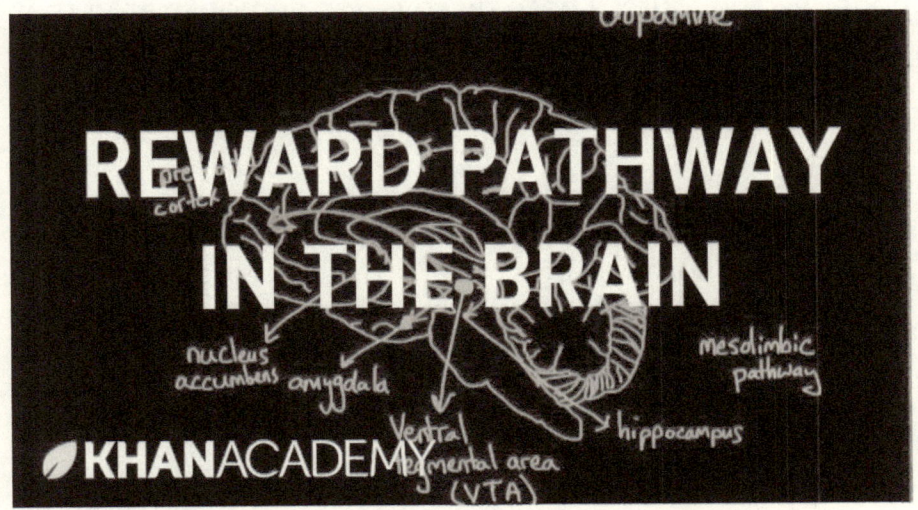

The Biology of Reward

The pleasure and reward system in the brain was discovered by accident in 1954. The American psychologist James Olds was studying the rat brain's alerting process, when he mistakenly placed the electrodes in a part of the limbic system, a group of structures deep within the brain that are generally believed to play a role in emotions.

When the brain was wired so that the animal could stimulate this area by pressing a lever, Olds found that the rats would press the lever almost nonstop, as many as 5,000 times an hour. The animals would stimulate themselves to the exclusion of everything else except sleep. They would even endure tremendous pain and hardship for an opportunity to press the lever. Olds had clearly found an area in the limbic system that provided a powerful reward for these animals.

Research on human subjects revealed that the electrical stimulation of some areas of the brain (the medial hypothalamus) produced a feeling of quasi-orgasmic sexual arousal (Olds and Olds 1969). If certain other areas of the brain were stimulated, an individual experienced a type of lightheadedness that banished negative thoughts. These discoveries demonstrated that pleasure is a distinct neurological function that is linked to a complex reward and reinforcement system (Hall, Bloom and Olds 1977).

During the past several decades research on the biological basis of chemical dependency has been able to establish some of the brain regions and neurotransmitters involved in reward. In particular it appears that the dependence on alcohol, opiates and cocaine relies on a common set of biochemical mechanisms (Cloninger 1983, Blum et al. 1989).

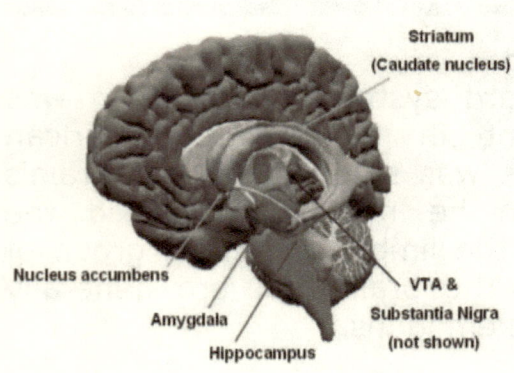

A neuronal circuit deep in the brain involving the limbic system and two regions called the nucleus accumbens and the globus pallidus appears to be critical in the expression of reward for people taking these drugs (Wise and Bozarth 1984). Although each substance of abuse appears to act on different parts of this circuit, the end result is the same: Dopamine is released in the nucleus accumbens and the hippocampus (Koob and Bloom 1988). Dopamine appears to be the primary neurotransmitter of reward at these reinforcement sites.

Although the system of neurotransmitters involved in the biology of reward is complex, at least three other neurotransmitters are known to be involved at several sites in the brain: serotonin in the hypothalamus, the enkephalins (opioid peptides) in the ventral tegmental area and the nucleus accumbens, and the inhibitory neurotransmitter GABA in the ventral tegmental area and the nucleus accumbens (Stein and Belluzi 1986, Blum 1989).

Interestingly, the glucose receptor is an important link between the serotonergic system and the opioid peptides in the hypothalamus. An alternative reward pathway involves the release of norepinephrine in the hippocampus from neuronal fibers that originate in the locus coeruleus. In a normal person, these neurotransmitters work together in a cascade of excitation or inhibition-between complex stimuli and complex responses-leading to a feeling of well being, the ultimate reward (Cloninger 1983, Stein and Belluzi 1986, Blum and Koslowski 1990).

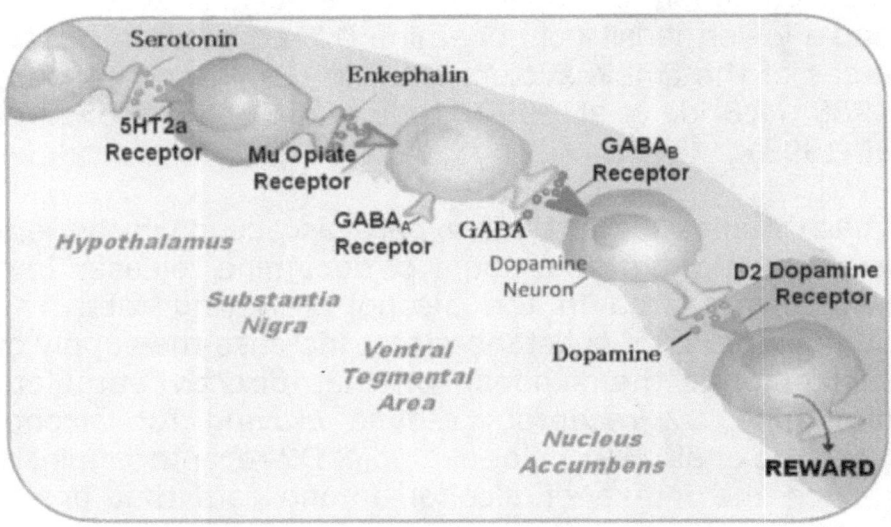

In **the cascade theory of reward**, a disruption of these intercellular interactions results in anxiety, anger and other "bad feelings" or in a craving for a substance that alleviates these negative emotions. Alcohol, for example, is known to activate the norepinephrine system in the limbic circuitry through an intercellular cascade that includes serotonin, opioid peptides and dopamine. Alcohol may also act directly through the production of neuroamines that interact with opioid receptors or with dopaminergic systems (Alvaksinen et al. 1984; Blum and Kozlowski 1990).

In the cascade theory of reward, genetic anomalies, prolonged stress or long-term abuse of alcohol can lead to a self-sustaining pattern of abnormal cravings in both animals and human beings.

Support for the cascade theory can be derived from a series of experiments on strains of rats that prefer alcohol to water. Compared to normal rats, the alcohol-preferring rats have fewer serotonin neurons in the hypothalamus, higher levels of enkephalin in the hypothalamus (because less is released), more GABA neurons in the nucleus accumbens (which inhibit the release of dopamine), a reduced supply of dopamine in the nucleus accumbens and a lower density of dopamine D2 receptors in certain areas of the limbic system (Russell, Lanin and Taljaard 1988; McBride et al. 1990; Zhou et al. 1990; McBride et al. 1993).

These studies suggest a four-part cascade in which there is a reduction in the amount of dopamine released in a key reward area in the alcohol-preferring rats. The administration of substances that increase the supply of serotonin at the synapse or that directly stimulate dopamine D2 receptors reduce craving for alcohol (McBride et al. 1993). For example, D2 receptor agonists reduce the intake of alcohol among rats that prefer alcohol, whereas D2 dopamine-receptor antagonist increase the drinking of alcohol in these inbred animals (Dyr et al. 1993).

Support for the cascade theory of alcoholism in human beings is found in a series of clinical trials. When amino-acid precursors of certain neurotransmitters (serotonin and dopamine) and a drug that promotes enkephalin activity were given to alcoholic subjects, the individuals experienced fewer cravings for alcohol, a reduced incidence of stress, an increased likelihood of recovery and a reduction in relapse rates (Brown et al. 1990; Blum and Tractenberg 1988; Blum, Briggs and Tractenberg 1989).

Furthermore, the notion that dopamine is the "final common pathway" for drugs such as cocaine, morphine and alcohol is supported by recent studies by Jordi Ortiz and his associates at Yale University School of Medicine and the University of Connecticut Health Services Center. These authors demonstrated that the chronic use of cocaine, morphine or alcohol results in several biochemical adaptations in the limbic dopamine system. They suggest that these adaptations may result in changes in the structural and functional properties of the dopaminergic system.

We believe that the biological substrates of reward that underlie the addiction to alcohol and other drugs are also the basis for impulsive, compulsive and addictive disorders comprising the reward deficiency syndrome.

Alcoholism and Genes
An alteration in any of the genes that are involved in the expression of the molecules in the reward cascade might predispose an individual to alcoholism. Indeed, the evidence for a genetic basis to alcoholism has accumulated steadily over the past five decades. The earliest report comes from studies of laboratory mice by the American psychologist L. Mirone in 1952.

Mirone found that, given a choice, certain mice preferred alcohol to water. Gerald McLearn at the University of California at Berkeley took this a step farther by producing an inbred mouse (the C57 strain) that had a marked preference for alcohol. The alcohol-preferring C57 strain bred true through successive generations-it was the first clear indication that alcoholism has a genetic basis (McLearn and Rodgers 1959).

The first evidence that alcoholism has a genetic basis in human beings came in 1972 when scientists at the Washington University School of Medicine in St. Louis found that adopted children whose biological parents were alcoholics were more likely to have a drinking problem than those born to nonalcoholic parents (Schuckit, Goodwin and Winokur 1972).

In 1973 Goodwin and Winokur, working at the Psykologisk Institut in Copenhagen, studied 5,483 men in Denmark who had been adopted in early childhood. They found that the sons born to alcoholic fathers were three times more likely to become alcoholic than the sons of nonalcoholic fathers.

In the late 1980s research on the inheritance of alcoholism suggested that there might be important genetic differences between alcoholics and nonalcoholics (Cloninger, Bohman and Sigvardsson 1981; Goodwin 1979). One of us (Blum) and his colleagues suspected that the activity of the chemical signaling molecules in the reward pathways of the brain might be involved.

Over the course of two years we compared eight genetic markers associated with various neurotransmitters (including serotonin, endogenous opioids, GABA, transferrin, acetylcholine, alcohol dehydrogenase and aldehyde dehydrogenase). In each instance we failed to find a direct association between the genetic markers and alcoholism.

The opportunity to investigate a ninth genetic marker arose after Olivier Civelli of the Vollum Institute at Oregon University cloned and sequenced the gene for one form of the dopamine D2 receptor. The D2 receptor is one of at least five physiologically distinct dopamine receptors (Dl, D2, D3, D4 and D5) found on the synaptic membranes of neurons in the brain (Sibley and Monsma 1992).

Previous studies had established that D2 receptors are expressed in neurons within the cerebral cortex and the limbic system, including the nucleus accumbens, the amygdala and the hippocampus. Because these are the same areas of the brain (with the exception of the cortex) that are believed to be involved in the reward cascade, Civelli's work provided the opportunity to investigate an important molecular candidate for genetic aberrations among alcoholics.

The technique we used to distinguish between the D2 receptor genes of alcoholics and those of nonalcoholics relies on the detection of restriction-fragment-length polymorphisms (RFLPs). This approach involves the use of DNA-cutting enzymes (restriction endonucleases) that cleave the DIMA molecule at specific nucleotide sequences. If there are genetic differences between two individuals such that a restriction enzyme cuts their DNA along different points in (or near) a gene, the resulting fragments of their genes will be of different lengths.

These differing fragments, or polymorphisms, are recognized by the use of a radioactivity labeled DNA probe-in this case a short sequence of the D2 receptor gene-that binds to a complementary DNA sequence on the fragments. Radio labeled fragments of different lengths signify a difference in the cleavage sequence recognized by the restriction enzyme (Grandy et al. 1989).

The restriction enzyme (Taq 1) cuts the nucleotide sequence at a site just outside the coding region for the D2 receptor gene. This produces the Taq 1A polymorphisms. To date there are four Taq 1A alleles known, the Al, A2, A3 and A4 alleles. The A3 and A4 alleles are rare, whereas the A2 allele is found in nearly 75 percent of the general population and the Al allele in about 25 percent of the population.

In 1990 we used the Taq I enzyme to search for Taq IA polymorphisms in the DNA extracted from the brains of deceased alcoholics and a control population of nonalcoholics. The results were striking: In our sample of 35 alcoholics we found that 69 percent had the Al allele and 31 percent had the A2 allele. In 35 nonalcoholics we found that 20 percent had the A1 allele and 80 percent had the A2 allele.

Since our 1990 study, some laboratories have failed to find a connection between the A1 allele and alcoholism. However, a review of their work shows that their samples were not limited to severe forms of alcoholism, which we believe to be an important distinguishing criterion. In our original study, over 70 percent of the alcoholics had cirrhosis of the liver, a disease suggestive of severe and chronic alcoholism. Moreover, the negative studies failed to adequately assess controls to eliminate alcoholism, drug abuse and other related "reward behaviors."

In this regard, Katherine Neiswanger and Shirley Hill of the University of Pittsburgh recently found a strong association of the A1 allele and alcoholism and suggested that early failures were the result of poor assessment of a true phenotype in the controls (Neiswanger, Kaplan and Hill 1995).

To date, 14 independent laboratories have supported the finding that the A1 allele is a causative factor in severe forms of alcoholism, though perhaps not in milder forms (Blum and Noble 1994). These findings do not prove that the A1 allele of the dopamine D2 receptor gene is the only cause of severe alcoholism, but they are a powerful indication that the A1 allele is involved with alcoholism.

Further evidence for the role of biology in alcoholism comes from efforts to find electrophysiological markers that might indicate a predisposition to the addictive disorder. One such marker is the latency and the magnitude of the positive 300-millisecond (P300) wave, an indicator of the general electrical activity of the brain that is evoked by a specific stimulus such as a tone.

It turns out that abnormalities in the electrical activity of the brain are evident in the young sons of alcoholic fathers. Their P300 waves are markedly reduced in amplitude compared to the P300 waves of the sons of nonalcoholic fathers. These results raised the question as to whether this deficit had been transferred from father to son and whether this deficit would predispose the son to substance abuse in the future (Begleiter, Porjexa, Bihari and Kissin 1984).

Experiments carried out since then have answered both questions. The alcoholic fathers had the same P300-wave deficit seen in their sons, and the sons showed increased drug-seeking behaviors (including alcohol and nicotine) compared to the sons of nonalcoholic fathers. Moreover, the sons of alcoholic fathers had an atypical neurocognitive profile (Whipple, Parker and Noble 1988).

It now appears that children with P300 abnormalities are more likely to abuse drugs and tobacco in later years (Berman, Whipple, Fitch and Noble 1993).

Remarkably, Noble and his colleagues found an association between the A1 allele and a prolonged latency of the P300 wave in children of alcoholics (Noble et al. 1994). Two of us (Blum and Braverman) extended this work and observed a similar correlation between the Al allele and a prolonged P300 latency in a neuropsychiatric population. Subjects who are homozygous for the Al allele showed significantly prolonged P300 latency compared to A1/A2 and A2/A2 carriers.

Drug Addiction and Smoking

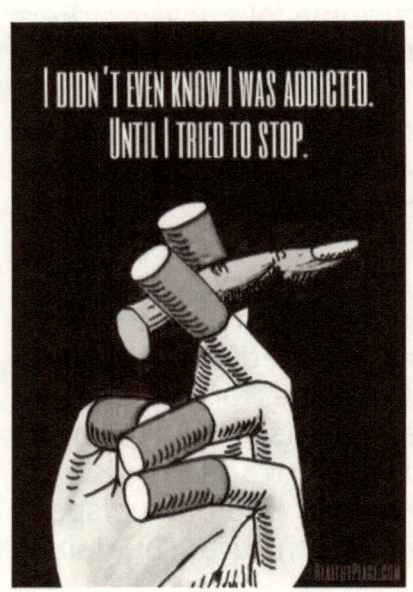

Cocaine can bring intense, but temporary, pleasure to the user. The aftermath is addiction and severe psychological and physiological harm. Various psychosocial theories have been advanced to account for the abuse of cocaine and other illicit drugs. In contrast to alcoholism, where growing empirical evidence is implicating hereditary factors, relatively little has been known about the genetics of human cocaine dependence.

However, some recent studies have suggested that hereditary factors are involved in the use and abuse of cocaine and other illicit drugs.

Studies of adopted children, for example, show that a biological background of alcohol problems in the parents predicts an increased tendency toward illicit drug abuse in the children (Cadoret, Froughton, O'Gorman and Heywood 1986). Similarly, family studies of cocaine addicts show a high percentage of first- or second-degree relatives who have been diagnosed as alcoholics (Miller, Gold, Belkin and Klaher 1989; Wallace 1990).

Behavioral anomalies such as conduct disorder (in which children violate social norms and the rights of others) and antisocial personality (the adult equivalent of conduct disorder) are often found to be associated with alcohol and drug problems. Several investigators have noted that sociopathic behavior in children predicts a tendency toward antisocial personality behavior, alcohol abuse and drug problems later in life. An analysis of 40 studies showed a strong positive correlation between alcoholism and drug abuse, between alcoholism and antisocial personality, and between drug abuse and antisocial personality (Schubert et al. 1988).

Although there is little known about the genetics of cocaine dependence, extensive scientific data are available on the effects of cocaine on brain chemistry. The current view is that the system that uses dopamine in the brain plays an important role in the pleasurable effects of cocaine. In animals, for example, the principal location where cocaine takes effect is the dopamine D2 receptor gene on chromosome 11 (Koob and Bloom 1988).

Recently George Koob and his colleagues of the Scripps Research Institute in La Jolla, California, found evidence suggesting that the dopamine D3 receptor gene is a primary site of cocaine effects. The exact effect of cocaine on gene expression is unknown. However, we do know that D2 receptors are decreased by chronic cocaine administration, and this may induce severe craving for cocaine and possibly cocaine dreams (Volkow et al. 1993).

A recent study by Ernest Noble of the University of California at Los Angeles and Blum found that about 52 percent of cocaine addicts have the Al allele of the dopamine D2 receptor gene, compared to only 21 percent of non addicts. The prevalence of the Al allele increases significantly with three risk factors: parental alcoholism and drug abuse; the potency of the cocaine used by the addict (intra nasal versus "crack" cocaine); and early-childhood deviant behavior, such as conduct disorder.

In fact, if the cocaine addict has three of these risk factors, the prevalence of the Al allele rises to 87 percent. These findings suggest that childhood behavioral disorders may signal a genetic predisposition to drug or alcohol addiction (Noble et al. 1993).

A recent survey by the National Institute of Drug Abuse of five independent studies showed that the Al allele is also associated with polysubstance dependence (Uhl, Blum, Noble and Smith 1993). The Al allele is also associated with an increase in the amount of money spent for drugs by polysubstance-dependent people (Comings et al. 1994).

Although not viewed in the same light as the use of cocaine and other illicit drugs, cigarette smoking is another form of chemical addiction. Most attempts to stop smoking are associated with withdrawal symptoms typical of the other chemical addictions. Although environmental factors may be important determinants of cigarette use, there is strong evidence that the acquisition of the smoking habit and its persistence are strongly influenced by hereditary factors.

Of particular significance are studies of identical twins, which show that when one twin smokes, the other tends to smoke. This is not the case in non identical twins. In one twin study, Dorit Carmelli of the Stanford Research Institute and her associates examined a national sample of male twins who were veterans of World War II.

A unique aspect of this study was that the twins were surveyed twice, once in 1967-68 and again 16 years later. This allowed an examination of genetic factors in all aspects of smoking-initiation, maintenance and quitting. In general, whatever happened to one identical twin happened to the other-including the long-term pattern of not smoking, smoking and then quitting smoking. The absence of these similarities in a control population of non-identical twins suggests a strong biogenetic component in smoking behavior (Swan et al. 1990).

Animal studies have suggested that the dopaminergic pathways of the brain may be involved. For example, the administration of nicotine to rodents disturbs dopamine metabolism in the reward centers of the brain to a greater extent than does the administration of alcohol.

With this in mind, one of us (Comings) and his colleagues investigated the incidence of the A1 allele in a population of Caucasian smokers. These smokers did not abuse alcohol or other drugs, but had made at least one unsuccessful attempt to stop smoking. It turned out that 48 percent of the smokers carried the A1 allele. The higher the prevalence of the A1 allele, the earlier had been the age of onset of smoking, the greater the amount of smoking and the greater the difficulty experienced in attempting to stop smoking.

In another sample of Caucasian smokers and nonsmokers, Noble and his colleagues found that the prevalence of the A1 allele was highest in current smokers, lower in those who had stopped smoking and lowest in those who had never smoked (Noble et al. 1994).

Compulsive Binging and Gambling

Obesity is a disease that comes in many forms. Once thought to be p r i m a r i l y environmental, it is now considered to have both genetic and environmental components. In a Swedish adoption study, for example, the weight of the adult adoptees was strongly 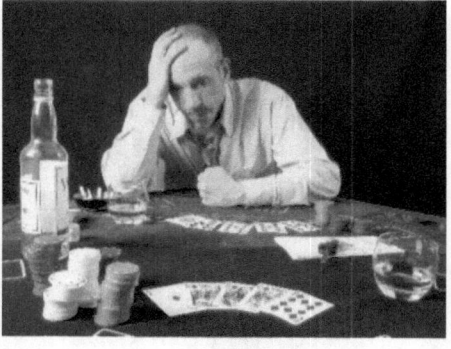 related to the body mass index of the biological parents and to the body-mass index of the adoptee parents. The links to both genetic and environmental factors were dramatic.

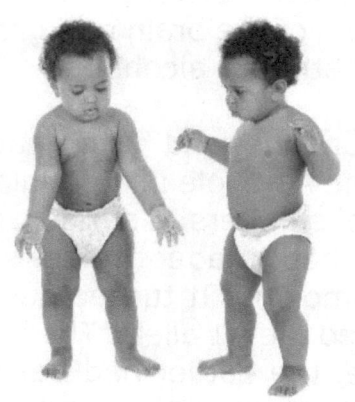

Other studies of adoptees and twins suggest that heredity is an important contributor to the development of obesity, whereas childhood environment has little or no influence. Moreover, the distribution of fat around the body has also been found to have heritable elements.

The inheritance of subcutaneous fat distribution is genetically separable from body fat stored in other compartments (among the viscera in the abdomen, for example). It has been suggested that there is evidence for both single and multiple gene anomalies (Bouchard 1995).

Given the complex array of metabolic systems that contribute to overeating and obesity, it is not surprising that a number of neurochemical defects have been implicated. Indeed at least three such genes have been found: one associated with cholesterol production, one with fat transport and one related to insulin production (Bouchard 1995). The ob gene and its product the leptin protein have also been implicated in regulating long-term eating behavior (Zhang et al. 1994).

Most recently another protein, glucagon-like peptide 1 (GLP-1) has been found to be involved in the regulation of short-term eating behavior (Turton et al. 1996). The relationship between leptin and GLP-1 is not known. The ob gene may be involved in the animal's selection of fat, but perhaps not in the ingestion of carbohydrates, which appears to be regulated by the dopaminergic system. It may be that the ob gene is functionally linked to the opioid peptodergic systems involved in reward.

Whatever the relation between these systems, the complexity of compulsive eating disorders suggests that more than one defective gene is involved. Indeed, the relation between compulsive overeating and drug and alcohol addiction is well documented (Krahn 1991, Newman and Gold 1992). Neurochemical studies show that pleasure-seeking behavior is a common denominator of addiction to alcohol, drugs and carbohydrates (Blum et al. 1990).

Alcohol, drugs and carbohydrates all cause the release of dopamine in the primary reward area of the brain, the nucleus accumbens. Although the precise localization and specificity of the pleasure-inducing properties of alcohol, drugs and food are still debated, there is general agreement that they work through the dopaminergic pathways of the brain. Other studies suggest the involvement of at least three other neurotransmitters serotonin, GABA and the opioid peptides.

Variants of the dopamine D2 receptor gene appear to be risk factors in obesity. The Al allele was present in 45 percent of obese subjects as compared to 19 percent of non-obese subjects (Noble, Noble and Ritchie 1994). Furthermore, the Al allele was not associated with a number of other metabolic and cardiovascular risks, including elevated levels of cholesterol and high blood pressure.

In contrast, when the subject's profile included factors such as parental obesity, a later onset of obesity and carbohydrate preference, the prevalence of the Al allele rose to 85 percent. More recently another study found a significant association between genetic variants of the D2 receptor and obese subjects (Comings et al. 1993).

There is also an increased prevalence of the Al allele in obese subjects who have severe alcohol and drug dependence (Blum et al. 1996a).

When obesity, alcoholism and drug addiction were found in a patient, the incidence of the Al allele rose to 82 percent. In contrast, the allele had an incidence of zero percent in non-obese patients who were also not substance abusers and did not have a family history of substance abuse. The presence of the dopamine D2 receptor gene variants increases the risk of obesity and related behaviors.

Pathological gambling-in which an individual becomes obsessed with the act of risking money or possessions for greater "payoffs" occurs at a rate of less than two percent in the general population. Although it is the most socially acceptable of the behavioral addictions, pathological gambling has many affinities to alcohol and drug abuse.

Clinicians have remarked on the similarity between the aroused euphoric state of the gambler and the "high" of the cocaine addict or substance abuser. Pathological gamblers express a distinct craving for the "feel" of gambling; they develop tolerance in that they need to take greater risks and make larger bets to reach a desired level of excitement, and they experience withdrawal-like symptoms (anxiety and irritability) when no "action" is available (Volberg and Steadman 1988).

Indeed, there is a typical course of progression through four stages of the compulsive-gambling syndrome winning, losing, desperation and hopelessness-a series not uncommon to other addictive behaviors.

Might the dopamine pathways in the brain be involved with pathological gambling? A recent study of Caucasian pathological gamblers found that 50.9 percent carried the A1 allele of the dopamine D2 receptor (Comings et al. 1996b). The more severe the gambling problem, the more likely it was that the individual was a carrier of the Al allele.

Finally, in a population of males with drug problems who were also pathological gamblers the incidence of the Al allele rose to 76 percent.

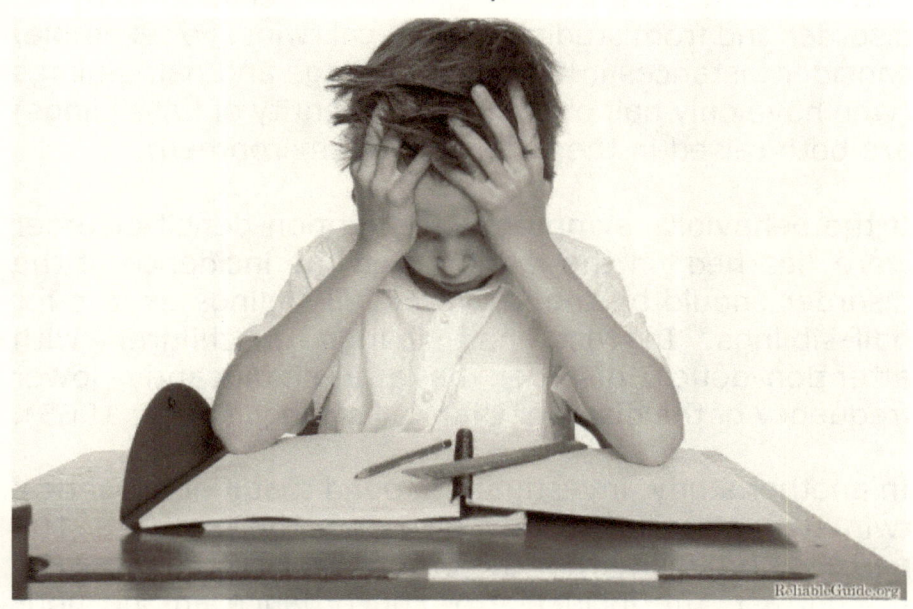

Attention-Deficit Disorder

This disorder is most commonly found among school-age boys, who are at least four times more likely to express the symptoms than are young girls. These children have difficulty applying themselves to tasks that require a sustained mental effort, they can be easily distracted, they may have difficulty remaining seated without fidgeting and they may impulsively blurt out answers in the classroom or fail to wait their turn. Although normal children occasionally display these symptoms, attention-deficit disorder is diagnosed when the behavior's persistence and severity impedes the child's social development and education.

Early speculation about the causes of attention-deficit disorder focused on potential sources of stress within the child's family, including marital discord, poor parenting, psychiatric illness, alcoholism or drug abuse. It has become progressively clear, however, that stress within the family cannot explain the incidence of the disorder.

There is now little doubt that the disorder has a genetic basis. Evidence in support of this notion comes from patterns of inheritance in the families of children with the disorder and from studies of identical twins. For example, consider instances in which full siblings and half-siblings (who have only half of the genetic identity of full siblings) are both raised in the same family environment.

If the behavioral symptoms of attention-deficit disorder were "learned" in the family, then the incidence of the disorder should be the same for full siblings as it is for half-siblings. In fact, half-siblings of children with attention-deficit disorder have a significantly lower frequency of the disorder than full siblings (Lopez 1965).

In another study, investigators found that if one identical twin had attention-deficit disorder, there was a 100 percent probability that the other also had the disorder. In contrast, the incidence of concordance among non-identical twins was only 17 percent. This result has been supported by two other independent studies of identical twins (Willerman 1973).

Finally, one of us (Comings) and his coworkers found that the A1 allele of the dopamine D2 receptor gene was present in 49 percent of the children with attention-deficit disorder compared to only 27 percent of the controls (Comings et al. 1991).

Some other recent work has linked attention-deficit disorder with another impulsive disorder: Tourette syndrome. More than 100 years ago the French neurologist Giles de la Tourette described a condition that was characterized by compulsive swearing, multiple muscle tics and loud noises. He found that the disorder usually appeared in children between 7 to 10 years old, with boys more likely to be affected than girls. Tourette suggested that the condition might be inherited.

In the early 1980s one of us (Comings) and his colleagues studied 246 families in which at least one member of the family had Tourette disorder. The study indicated that virtually all cases of Tourette syndrome are genetic (Comings et al. 1991). Subsequent studies also found that there was a high incidence of impulsive, compulsive, addictive, mood and anxiety disorders on both sides of the affected individual's family (Comings and Comings 1987).

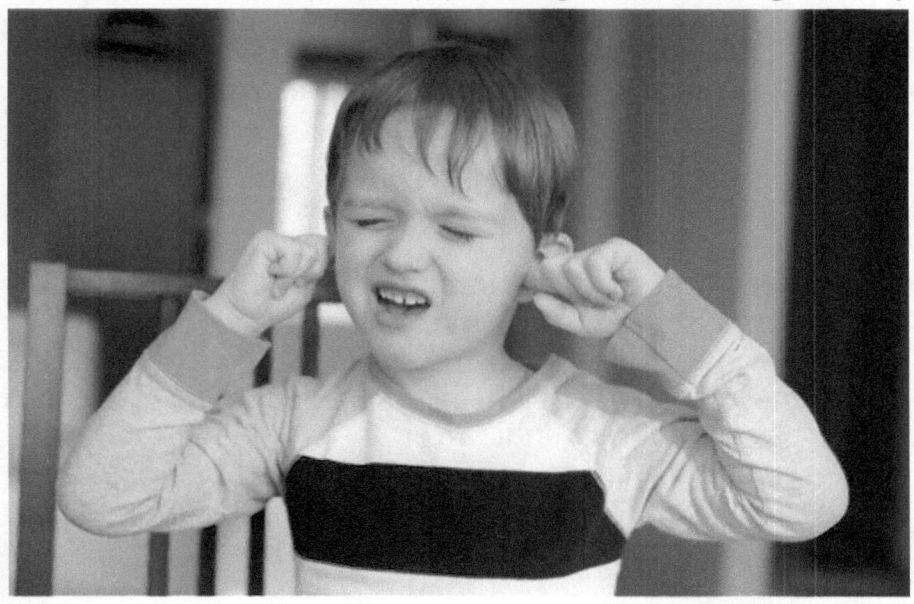

The Al allele was implicated in a recent report showing that nearly 45 percent of the people diagnosed with Tourette disorder carried the aberrant gene (Comings et al. 1991). Moreover, the Al allele had the highest incidence among people who had the severest manifestations of the disorder.

As mentioned earlier, Tourette syndrome appears to be tightly coupled to attention-deficit disorder. In studies of the two disorders, it was found that 50 to 80 percent of the people with Tourette syndrome also had attention-deficit disorder. Furthermore, an increased number of relatives of individuals with Tourette disorder also had attention-deficit/hyperactivity disorder (Knell & Commings)

It now appears that Tourette syndrome is a complex illness that may include attention-deficit disorder, conduct disorder, obsessive, compulsive and addictive disorders and other related disorders. The close coupling between these disorders has led one of us (Comings) to propose that Tourette syndrome is a severe form of attention-deficit disorder (Comings and Comings 1989; Comings 1995).

The high frequency of the Al allele among people with Tourette syndrome and attention-deficit disorder raises the question of whether other genes affecting dopaminergic function might also be involved in these Disorders.

Two others that have been considered are the gene for the enzyme dopamine B-hydroxylase, which converts dopamine to norepinephrine, and the gene for the dopamine transporter, which takes dopamine back into the presynaptic terminal after it is released into the synapse. In both cases, variant forms of these genes are associated with Tourette syndrome (Comings et al. 1996c).

The anomalous dopamine B-hydroxylase gene (the "DBH Taq BI" allele) was further associated with learning disabilities, conduct disorder and substance abuse, whereas the variant of the dopamine transporter (the "10 repeat" allele) was also associated with alcohol abuse, depression and obsessive-compulsive disorder.

This observation was supported by other work showing that the 10 repeat allele for the dopamine transporter gene was associated with attention-deficit/hyperactivity disorder (Cook et al. 1995). Moreover, elevated levels of the dopamine transporter molecule have been found in the brains of patients with Tourette syndrome (Malison et al. 1995).

If these dopamine-related molecules are indeed associated with various behavioral disorders, it might be expected that having more than one variant would increase the severity or the likelihood of having a disorder. Indeed, this is the case: The severity of attention-deficit disorder, conduct disorder, substance abuse and mood disorders progressively increased from individuals carrying none of the genes to those who carried all three genes (Comings et al. 1996c).

Given the widespread prevalence of attention-deficit disorder among children, and its frequent association with alcoholism, drug dependence and other behavioral disorders, it may be that childhood attention-deficit disorder is a predisposing cause to various disorders among adults. For example, there is a significant correlation between attention-deficit hyperactivity disorder and adult drug abuse (Gittleman, Mannuzza, Shenker and Bonagura 1985).

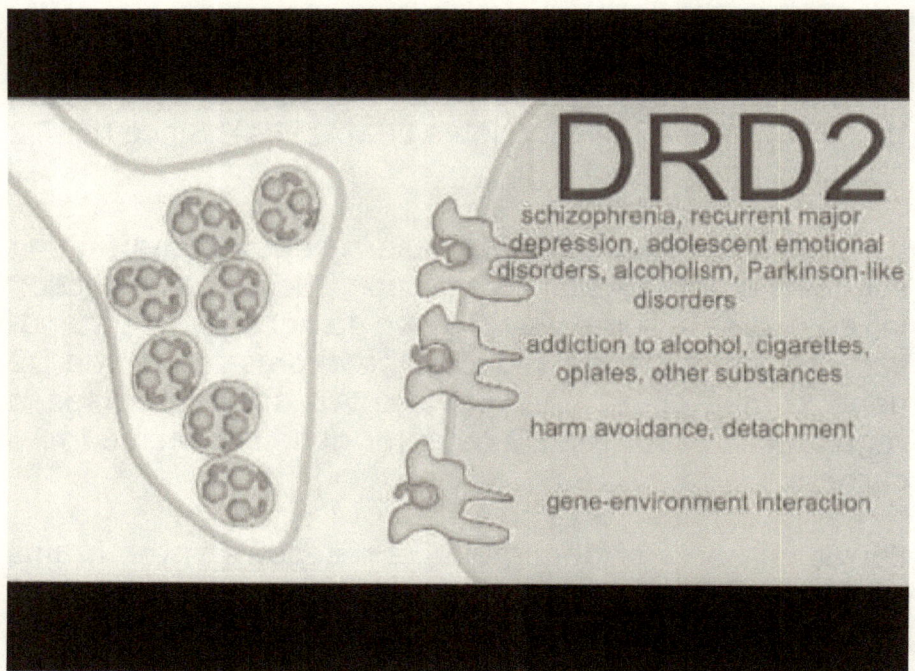

The Dopamine D2 Receptor

The Al allele carries a behavioral risk factor that shows up not only in substance addiction and attention-deficit disorder, but also in antisocial behavior, conduct disorder and violent or aggressive behavior. In a recent study the Al allele was present in 60 percent of a sample population of young adolescents between 12 and 18 years old who were diagnosed as "pathologically violent" subjects (Blum Unpublished).

A variant of the dopamine transporter gene (VENT 10 repeat) was present in 100 percent of the adolescents. Of these 70 percent had the so-called 10/10 form whereas 30 percent carried the 10/9 allelic form. Another study found that 59 percent of Vietnam veterans with Posttraumatic stress disorder also carried the Al allele, compared to only 5 percent of veterans who were exposed to similar stress but did not develop the disorder (Comings, Muhleman and Gysin 1996).

Why would carriers of the Al allele be predisposed to the spectrum of disorders associated with the reward deficiency syndrome? Individuals having the Al allele have approximately 30 percent fewer D2 receptors than those with the A2 allele (Noble et al. 1991). Since the D2 receptor gene

controls the production of these receptors, the finding suggests that the A1 allele is responsible for the reduction in receptors. In some way that we do not yet understand, carrying the A1 allele reduces the expression of the D2 gene compared to carrying the A2 allele. Perhaps a regulatory site for the D2 receptor gene is affected in A1 carriers.

Fewer numbers of dopamine D2 receptors in the brains of A1 allele carriers may translate into lower levels of dopaminergic activity in those parts of the brain involved in reward. A1 carriers may not be sufficiently rewarded by stimuli that A2 carriers find satisfying. This may translate into the persistent cravings or stimulus-seeking behavior of A1 carriers. Moreover, because dopamine is known to reduce stress, individuals who carry the A1 allele may have difficulty coping with the normal pressures of life. In response to stress or cravings, A1 carriers may turn to other substances or activities that release additional quantities of dopamine in an attempt to gain temporary relief.

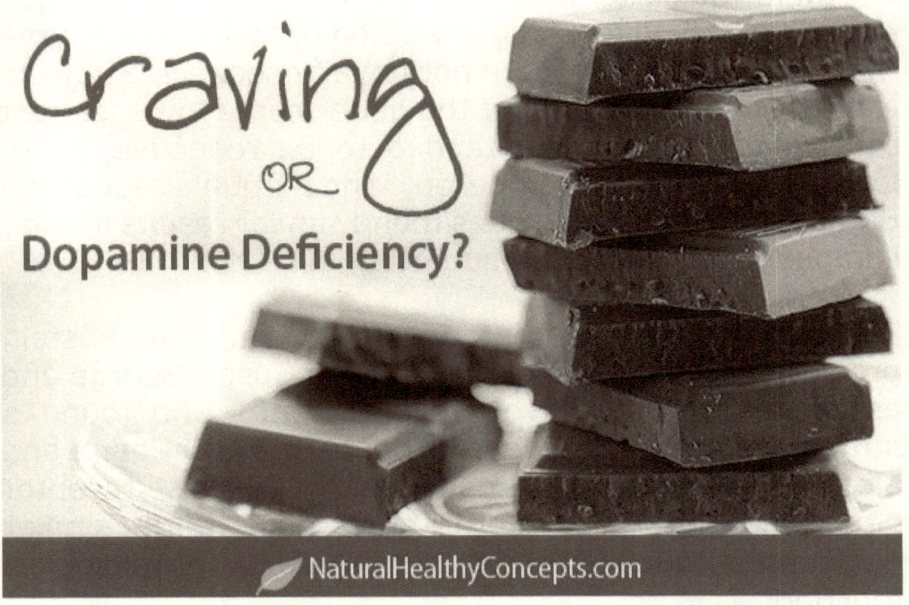

Craving OR

Dopamine Deficiency?

NaturalHealthyConcepts.com

Alcohol, cocaine, marijuana, nicotine and carbohydrates (like chocolate) all cause the release of dopamine in the brain and bring about a temporary relief of craving. These substances can be used singly, in combination or to some extent interchangeably. Although we believe that the gene for the D2 receptor plays a critical role in reward deficiency syndrome, other genes (such as the dopamine transporter gene) are undoubtedly involved in the different manifestations of the syndrome.

Scientists from Israel and the National Institute of Mental Health recently showed that a genetic variation of the dopamine D4 receptor gene is associated with people who are novelty (or sensation) seekers (Ebstein et al.

1996 and Benjamin et al. 1996). Both studies set out to test the hypothesis advanced by Robert Cloninger of Washington University that novelty-seeking behavior is modulated by the way brain cells process dopamine.

Richard Ebstein and his colleagues at the Herzog Memorial Hospital in Jerusalem found that novelty seekers-who tended to be compulsive, exploratory, fickle, excitable, quick-tempered and extravagant-were much more likely to have a longer version of the receptor gene than individuals who were not novelty seekers. Subjects with the shorter version of the gene scored lower on test of novelty seeking and tended to be reflective, rigid, loyal, stoic, slow-tempered and frugal. Jonathan Benjamin and his colleagues found similar results in their sample of 315 American subjects.

The work from the laboratories of Benjamin and Ebstein provide support of the earlier work of Susan George and associates at the University of Toronto who found a strong association between variants of the D4 gene and alcoholism and nicotine dependence. The D2 receptor gene and the D4 receptor gene have fairly similar nucleotide sequences and may have similar physiological functions.

In this respect, it is intriguing that investigators at the University of California, Los Angeles found an association between the A1 allele and individuals who were classified as "sensation seekers" and were characterized by agitation, impulsivity, excitability and a "hot temper" (Compton et al. unpublished). All of these studies further support a connection between the reward deficiency syndrome and the dopaminergic system.

Treatment
In the United States alone there are 18 million alcoholics, 28 million children of alcoholics, 6 million cocaine addicts, 14.9 million people who abuse other substances, 25

million people addicted to nicotine, 54 million people who are at least 20 percent overweight, 3.5 million school-age children with attention-deficit disorder or Tourette syndrome, and about 448,000 compulsive gamblers. We believe that recognizing the role of dopamine and the D2 receptor in the manifestation of these addictions and disorders is the first step toward rational treatment for a devastating problem in our society.

There is reason to believe that a pharmacological approach could help people with reward deficiency syndrome. It is tempting to speculate that the pharmacological sensitivity of alcoholics to dopaminergic agonists (bromocriptine, bupropion and n-propylnor-apomorphine) may be partly determined by the individual's D2 genotype.

We predict that Al carriers should be pharmacologically more responsive to D2 agonists, especially in the treatment of alcoholics or stimulant-dependent people. At least one study has already shown that the direct microinjection of the D2 agonist n-propylnor-apomorphine into the rat nucleus accumbens significantly suppresses the animal's symptoms after the withdrawal of opiates (Harris and Aston-Jones, 1994).

A recent double-blind study demonstrates the utility of this approach in human subjects (Lawford et al. 1995). The D2 agonist bromocryptine or a placebo was administered to alcoholics who were carriers of the Al allele (Al/Al and A1/A2 genotypes) or who only carried the A2 allele (A2/A2). The greatest improvement in the reduction of craving and anxiety was found among the Al carriers who were treated with bromocryptine. The attrition rate was highest among the Al carriers who were treated with the placebo.

These findings provide an important rationale for DNA testing to detect genetic variants for the D2 receptor or other dopamine-related genetic variants in the tertiary treatment of alcoholism. Unlike certain other complex disorders, such as Alzheimer's disease, the early identification and treatment of alcohol and drug abuse can occasionally alter the devastating course of these addictions.

Consider the successes of self-help programs such as Alcoholics Anonymous and Narcotics Anonymous, psychopharmacological adjunctive therapy, neuroregulation or brain-wave training and electrophysiological stimulation. Identifying individuals with the A1 allele offers the possibility of helping individuals before alcoholism or substance abuse affect their lives.

We foresee the possibility for better treatment, new forms of prevention and the removal of the social stigma attached not only to alcoholism but also to related "reward-seeking" behaviors comprising the reward deficiency syndrome.

Bibliography
Alvaksinen, M. N., V. Saano, H. Juvonene, A. Huhtikangas and J. Gunther. 1984. Binding of beta-carbolines and tetrahydroisoquinolines by opiate receptors of the d-type.

Acta Pharmacologica et Toxicologica 55:380-385.

Begleiter, H. B., Porjexa, B. Bihari and B. Kissin. 1984. Event-related brain potentials in boys at risk for alcoholism. Science 225:1493-1496.

Benjamin, J., L. Lin, C. Patterson, B. D. Greenberg, D. L. Murphy and D. H. Hamer. 1996. Population and familial association between the D4 dopamine receptor gene and measures of novelty seeking. Nature Genetics 12:81-84

Berman, S. M., S. C. Whipple, R. J. Fitch and E. P. Noble. 1993. P300 in boys as a predictor of adolescent substance use. Alcohol 10:69-76.

Blum, K. 1989. A commentary on neurotransmitter restoration as a common mode of treatment for alcohol, cocaine and opiate abuse. Integrative Psychiatry 6:199-204.

Blum, K., E. R. Braverman, R. G. Wood, J. Gill, C. Li, T. J. H. Chen, M. Taub, S. T. Montgomery, J. G. Cull and P. J. Sheridan. 1996a. Increase prevalence of the TaqI allele of the dopamine receptor gene (DRD2) in obesity with comorbid substance use disorder: preliminary findings. Pharmacogenetics (in press).

Blum, K., A. H. Briggs and M. C. Trachtenberg. 1989. Ethanol ingestive behavior as a function of central neurotransmission. Experientia 46:444-452.

Blum, K., and G. P. Kozlowski. 1990. Ethanol and neuromodulator interactions: a cascade model of reward. Progress in Alcohol Research 2:131-149.

Blum, K., and E. P. Noble. 1994. The sobering D2 story. Science 265:1346-1347.

Blum, K., E. P. Noble, P. J. Sheridan, A. Montgomery, T. Ritchie, P. Jagadeeswaran, H. Nogami, A. H. Briggs and J. B. Cohn. 1990. Allelic association of human dopamine D2 receptor gene in alcoholism. Journal of the American Medical Association 263:2055-2060.

Blum, K., P. 3. Sheridan, R. G. Wood, E. R. Braverman, T. J. H. Chen, J. G. Cull and D. E. Comings. 1996b. The D2 dopamine receptor gene as a predictor of reward deficiency syndrome: Bayes theorem. Journal of the Royal Society of Medicine (in press).

Blum, K., and Trachtenberg, M.C. 1988. Neurogenic deficits caused by alcoholism: restoration by SAAVE. Journal of Psychoactive Drugs 20:297-312.

Blum, K., M. C. Trachtenberg and D. W. Cook. 1990. Neuronutrient effects on weight loss in carbohydrate bingers: An open clinical trial. Current Therapeutic Research 48:217-233.

Blum, K., M. C. Trachtenberg, C. E. Elliott, M. L. Dingier, R. L. Sexton, A. I. Samuels and L. Cataldie. 1989. Enkephalinase inhibition and precursor amino acid loading improves inpatient treatment of alcohol and polydrug abusers: double-blind placebo-controlled study of the nutritional adjunct SAAVE. Alcohol 5:481-493.

Bouchard, C. 1995. Genetics of obesity: an update on molecular markers. International Journal of Obesity 19 (Supplement 3):S10-S13.

Brown, R. J., K. Blum and M. C. Trachtenberg. 1990. Neurodynamics of relapse prevention: a neuronutrient approach to outpatient DUI offenders. Journal of Psychoactive Drugs 22:173-187.

Cadoret, R. J., E. Froughton, T. O'Gorman and E. Heywood. 1986. An adoption study of genetic and environmental factors in drug abuse. Archives of General Psychiatry 43:1131-1136.

Cloninger, C. R., M. Bohman and S. Sigvardsson. 1981. Inheritance of alcohol abuse: cross-fostering analysis of adopted men. Archives of General Psychiatry 38: 861-868.

Cloninger, C. R. 1983. Genetic and environmental factors in the development of alcoholism. Journal of Psychiatric Treatment Evaluation 5:487-496.

Comings, D. E. 1990. Tourette Syndrome and Human Behavior. Duarte, Calif.: Hope Press. Comings, D. E. 1995. Tourette syndrome: A hereditary neuropsychiatric spectrum disorder. Annals of Clinical Psychiatry 6:235-247.

Comings, B. G., and D. E. Comings. 1987. A controlled study of Tourette syndrome. V. Depression and mania. American Journal of Human Genetics 41:804-821.

Comings, D. E., and B. G. Comings. 1989. A controlled family history study of Tourette syndrome I. Attention deficit hyperactivity disorder, learning disorders and dyslexia. Journal of Clinical Psychiatry Sl:275-280.

Comings, D. E., B. G. Comings, D. Muhleman, G. Deitz, B. Shahbahrami, D. Tast, E. Knell, P. Kocsis, R. Baumgarten, B. W. Kovacs, D. L. Levy, M. Smith, J. M. Kane, J. A. Lieberman, D. N. Klein, J. MacMurray, J. Tosk, J. Sverd, R. Gysin and S. Flanagan. 1991. The dopamine D2 receptor locus as a modifying gene in neuropsychiatric disorders. Journal of the American Medical Association 266:1793-1800.

Comings, E. E., L. Ferry, S. Bradshaw-Robinson, R. Burchette, C. Chiu and D. Muhleman. 1996a. The dopamine D2 receptor (DRD2) gene: A genetic risk factor in smoking. Pharmacogenetics (in press).

Comings, D. E., S. D. Flanagan, G. Dietz, D. Muhleman, E. Knell and R. Gysin. 1993. The dopamine D2 receptor (DRD2) as a major gene in obesity and height. Biochemical Medicine and Metabolic Biology 50:176-185.

Comings, D. E., D. Muhleman, C. Ahn, R. Gysin and S. D. Flanagan. 1994. The dopamine D2 receptor gene: A genetic risk factor in substance abuse. Drug and Alcohol Dependence 34:175-180.

Comings, D. E., D. Muhleman and R. Gysin. 1996. The dopamine D2 receptor (DRD2) gene in Posttraumatic stress disorder: A study and replication. Biological Psychiatry (in press).

Comings, D. E., R. J. Rosenthal, H. R. Leiseur, L. Rugle, D. Muhleman, C. Chiu, F. Dietz and R. Gane. 1996b. The molecular genetics of pathological gambling: The DRD2 gene. Pharmacogenetics (in press).

Comings, D. E., H. Wu, C. Chiu, R. H. Ring, R. Gade, C. Ahn, J. P. MacMurray, G. Deitz, D. Muhleman. 1996c. Polygenic inheritance of Tourette syndrome, stuttering, attention deficit hyperactivity, conduct and oppositional defiant disorder: The additive and subtractive effect of three dopaminergic genes-DRD2, DbetaH and DATA. American Journal of Medical Genetics (Neuropsychiatric Genetics) (in press).

Cook, E. H., M. A. Stein, M. D. Drajowsi, W. Cox, D. M. Olkon, J. E. Kieffer and B. L. Leventhal. 1995. Association of attention-deficit disorder and the dopamine transporter gene. American Journal of Human Genetics 56: 993-998.

Dyr, W., W. J. McBride, T. K. Lumeng, and J. M. Murphy. 1993. Effects of D1 and D2 dopamine receptor agents on ethanol consumption in the high-alcohol-drinking (HAD) line of rats. Alcohol 10:207-212.

Ebstein, R. P., O. Novick, R. Umansky, B. Priel, Y. Osher, D. Blaine, E. Bennett, L. Nemanov, M. Katz and R. Belmaker. (1996). Dopamine D4 receptor (D4DR) exon III polymorphism associated with the human personality trait of Novelty Seeking. Nature Genetics 12:78-80.

Gittelman, R., S. Mannuzza, R. Shenker and N. Bonagura. 1985. Hyperactive boys almost grown up. I. Psychiatric status. Archives of General Psychiatry 42:937-947.

Goodwin, D. S. 1979. Alcoholism and heredity. Archives of General Psychiatry 36: 57-61.

Grandy, D. K., M. Lih, L. Allen, J. R. Bunzow, M. Marchionni, H. Makam, L. Reed, R. E. Magenis and D. Civelli. 1989. The human dopamine D2 receptor gene is located on chromosome 11 at q22-q23 and identified as Taq I RLFP. American Journal of Human Genetics 45:778-785.

Hall, R. D., F. E. Bloom and J. Olds. 1977. Neuronal and neurochemical substrates of reinforcement. Neuroscience Research Program Bulletin 15:131-314.

Harris, G. C., and G. Aston-Jones. 1994. Involvement of D2 dopamine receptors in the nucleus accumbens in the opiate withdrawal syndrome. Nature 371(6493): 155-157.

Knell, E., and D. E. Comings. 1993. Tourette syndrome and attention deficit hyperactivity disorder: Evidence for a genetic relationship. Journal of Clinical Psychiatry 54:331-337.

Koob, G. F., and F. E. Bloom. 1988. Cellular and molecular mechanisms of drug dependence. Science 242:715-723.

Krahn, D. 1991. The relationship of eating disorders and substance abuse. Journal of Studies on Alcohol 3:239-253.

Lawford, B. R., R. M. Young, J. Rowell, J. Qualichefski, B. H. Fletcher, K. Syndulko, T. Ritchie and E. P. Noble. 1995. Bromocriptine in the treatment of alcoholics with the D2 dopamine receptor A1 allele. Nature Medicine 1:337-341.

Lopez, R. 1965. Hyperactivity in twins. Canadian Psychological Association 10:421-426.

McBride, W. J., X. M. Guan, E. Chernet, L. Lumeng and T.-K. Li. 1990. Regional differences in the densities of serotonin 1A receptors between P and NP rats. Alcoholism: Clinical and Experimental Research 14:316, abstract.

McBride, W. J., E. Chernet, W. Dyr, L. Lumeng and T.-K. Li. 1993. Densities of dopamine D2 receptors are reduced in CNS regions of alcohol preferring P rats. Alcohol 10:387-390.

McLearn, G. E., and D. A. Rodgers. 1959. Differences in alcohol preferences among inbred strains of mice. Quarterly Journal of Studies on Alcohol 20:691-695.

Malison, R. T., C. J. McDougle, C. H. van Dyck, L. Scahill, R. M. Baldwin, J. P. Seibyle, L. H. Price, J. F. Leckman and R. B. Innis. 1995. [123I]b-CIT SPECT imaging of striatal dopamine transporter binding in Tourette's disorder. American Journal of Psychiatry 152:1359-1361.

Miller, N. S., M. S. Gold, B. M. Belkin, A. L. Klaher. 1989. The diagnosis of alcohol and cannabis dependence in cocaine dependents and alcohol dependence in their families. British Journal of Addiction 84:1491-1498.

Neiswanger, K., B. B. Kaplan and S. Y. Hill. 1995. What can the DRD2/alcoholism story teach us about association studies in psychiatric genetics. American Journal of Medical Genetics (Neuropsychiatric Genetics) 60:272-275.

Newman, M. M, and M. S. Gold 1992. Preliminary findings of patterns of substance abuse in eating. American Journal of Drugs and Alcohol Abuse 18:207-211.

Noble, E. P., S. M. Berman and T. Z. Ozkaragoz. 1994. Prolonged P300 latency in children with the D2 dopamine receptor A1 allele. American Journal of Human Genetics 54:658-668.

Noble, E. P., K. Blum, M. E. Khalsa, T. Ritchie, A. Montgomery, R. C. Wood, R. J. Fitch, T. Ozkaragoz, P. J. Sheridan, M. D. Anglin, A. Paredes, L. J. Treiman and R. S. Sparks. 1993. Allelic association of the D2 dopamine receptor gene with cocaine dependence. Drug and Alcohol Dependence 83:271-285.

Noble, E. P. K. Blum, T. Ritchie, A. Montgomery and P. J. Sheridan. 1991. Allelic association of the D2 dopamine receptor gene with receptor binding characteristics in alcoholism. Archives of General Psychiatry 48:648-654.

Noble, E. P., S. T. Jeor, T. Ritchie, K. Syndulko, S. C. Jeor, R. J. Fitch, R. L. Brunner and R. S. Sparkes. 1994. D2 dopamine receptor gene and cigarette smoking: A reward gene? Medical Hypothesis 42:257-260.

Noble, E. P., R. E. Noble and T. Ritchie. 1994. D2 dopamine receptor gene and obesity. Journal of Eating Disorders 15:205-217.

Olds, M. E., and J. Olds. 1969. Effects of lesions in medical forebrain bundle on self-stimulation behavior. American Journal of Physiology 217:1253-1264.

Routtenberg, A. 1978. The reward system of the brain. Scientific American 239:154-165.
Russell, V. A., M. C. L. Lanin and J. F. Taljaard. 1988. Effect of ethanol on 3H-dopamine release in rat nucleus accumbens and striatal slices. Neurochemical Research 13:487-492.

Schubert, D. S. P., A. W. Wolf, M. B. Paterson, T. P. Grande and L. Pendleton. 1988. A statistical evaluation of the literature regarding the associations among alcoholism, drug abuse and antisocial personality disorder. International Journal of Addiction 23:797-808.

Schuckit, M. A., D. W. Goodwin and G. Winokur. 1972. A study of alcoholism in half-siblings. American Journal of Psychiatry 128:1132-1136.

Sibley, D., and F. J. Monsma. Molecular biology of dopamine receptors. 1992. Trends in Pharmacological Sciences 13:61-69.

Stein, L., and Belluzzi, J.D. 1986. Second messenger, natural rewards, and drugs of abuse. Clinical Neuropharmacology 9(Suppl. 4):205-209.

Swan, G. E., D. Carmelli, R. H. Rosenman, R. R. Fabsitz and J. C. Christian. 1990. Smoking and alcohol consumption in adult male twins: genetic heritability and shared environmental influence. Journal of Substance Abuse 2:39-50.

Turton, M. D., D. O'Shea, I. Gunn, S. A. Beak, C. M. B. Edwards, K. Meeran, S.J. Choi, G. M. Taylor, M. M. Heath, P. D. Lambert, J. P. H. Wilding, D. M. Smith, M. A. Gahel, J. Herbert, S. R. Bloom. 1996. A role for glucagon-like peptide-1 in the central regulation of feeding. Nature 379:60-72.

Uhl, G., K. Blum, E. P. Noble and S. Smith. 1993. Substance abuse vulnerability and D2 receptor genes. Trends in Neuroscience 16:83-88.

Volberg, R. A., and H. J. Steadman. 1988. Refining prevalence estimates of pathological gambling. American Journal of Psychiatry 145:502-505.

Volkow, N. D., J. S. Fowler, G.-J. Wang, R. Hitzemann, J. Logan, D. Schlyer, S. Dewey and A. P. Wolf. 1993. Decreased dopamine D2 receptor availability is associated with reduced frontal metabolism in cocaine abusers. Synapse 14:169-177.

Wallace, B. C. 1990. Crack cocaine smokers as adult children of alcoholics. The dysfunctional family link. Journal of Substance Abuse Treatment 7:89-100.

Whipple, S. C., E. S. Parker and E. P. Noble. 1988. An atypical neurocognitive profile in alcoholic fathers and their sons. Journal of Studies in Alcohol 49:240-244.

Willerman, L. 1973. Activity level and hyperactivity in twins. Child Development 44:288-293.

Wise, R. A., and M. A. Bozarth. 1984. Brain reward circuitry: four circuit elements "wired" in apparent series. Brain Research Bulletin 297:265-273.

Zhang, X., R. Proenca, M. Barone, L. Leopold, J. M. Friedman. 1994. Positional cloning of the mouse obese gene and its human homologue. Nature 372(6505):425-32.

Zhou, F. C., S. Bledsoe, L. Lumeng and T.-K. Li. 1990. Serotonergic immuno-stained terminal fibers are decreased in selected brain areas of alcohol-preferring P rats. Alcoholism: Clinical and Experimental Research 14:355, abstract.

@merican Scientist 1996 The Root of Reward of Reward Deficiency Syndrome Shah Aashna Hossain

"What has spawned a new way of looking at addiction is the fact that many of the potent motivational, and hence addictive, properties of different substances seem to involve a common neurochemical action: a "relationship between neurotransmitters, their receptors in the brain and addictive action."

Bozarth, director of the Addiction Research Unit in the Department of Psychology in the College of Arts and Letters.

In the Hebb laboratory of McGill University in 1954, research psychologist James Olds was running a series of experiments involving the neurological alerting process of rats. Accidentally, he placed some electrodes inside the rats' limbic system - a part of the brain containing a group of structures that play a role in emotions.

The brain was wired in a way that this area could be stimulated when the rat pressed on a lever. Curiously enough, the rats went back to pressing the connected lever time and time again - even up to 5,000 times per hour. They even denied themselves everything except sleep for the stimulation provided. Carried out in the medial hypothalamus region of human brains, this experiment was found to provide its subjects with feelings resembling orgasmic sexual arousal. And if certain other areas of the brain experienced stimulation, negative thoughts were eliminated and a feeling of lightheadedness would occur.

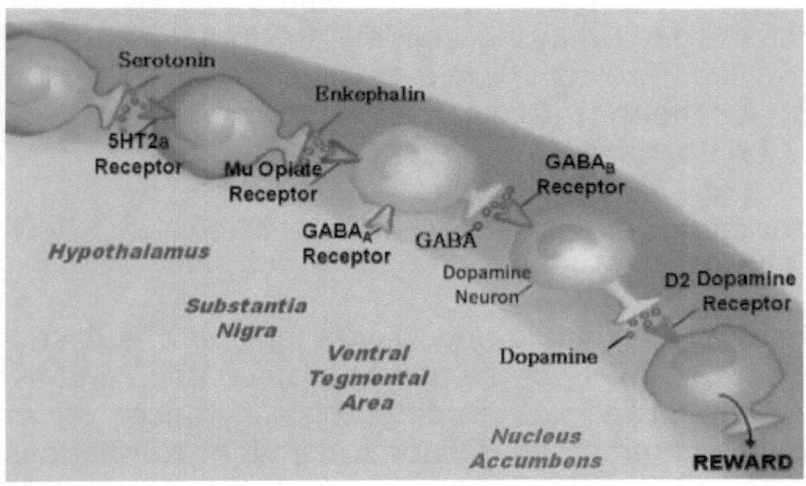

Thus was born the concept of the brain's reward pathway. In other words, the discovery that "pleasure is a distinct neurological function that is linked to a complex reward and reinforcement system".

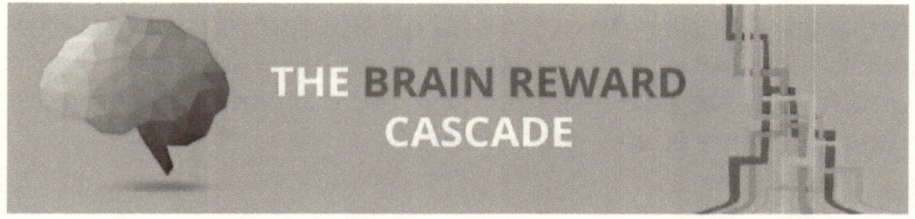

The Cascade Theory of Reward

Four regions of the brain and four neurotransmitters play a significant role and are a major part of the neurological reward pathway: dopamine in the nucleus accumbens and the hippocampus; serotonin in the hypothalamus; the enkephalins in the ventral tegmental area and the nucleus accumbens; GABA - an inhibitory neurotransmitter -also in the ventral tegmental area and the nucleus accumbens (Depression Despot, - link to map of the brain's limbic system) (3).

Out of all these neurotransmitters, dopamine has been singled out as "the primary neurotransmitter of reward." In the majority of people, the reward system begins with one of these chemicals spreading out to "network" and involve the other neurotransmitters in what resembles a cascade.
(http://www.sigmaxi.org/amsci/captions/captions96-03/blum-4.html - link to cascade system diagram) (3).

As a result, one feels "secure, calm, comfortable and satisfied," referred to as the "reward." In fact, a lot of research has shown that a significant amount of human behavior is aimed towards achieving such feelings. In its simplest definition, reward deficiency syndrome is what occurs when such "networking" does not occur (4).

Reward Deficiency Syndrome

Genetic abnormalities, exposure to a prolonged period of stress, and alcohol or other substance abuse leads to a corruption of the "cascade function" (3). Such a disruption in the interaction between the neurotransmitters results in the opposite of the "reward": feelings of anger, anxiety, and other emotions associated with negativity. It has also been linked with compulsive and impulsive disorders such as alcoholism and attention deficit hyperactivity disorder (5)

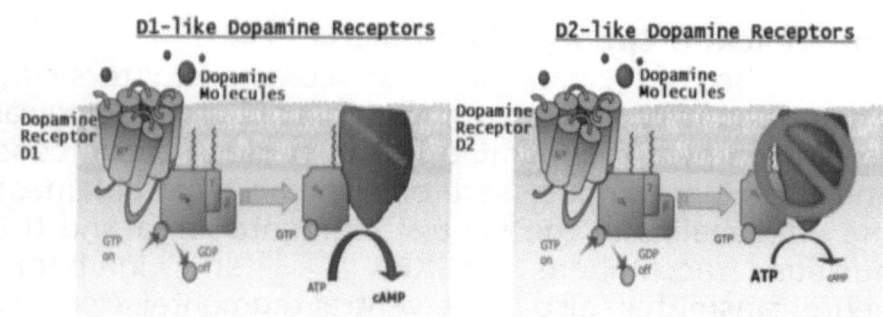

(http://www.sigmaxi.org/amsci/captions/captions96-03/blum-4.html - link to table of disorders associated with reward deficiency syndrome) (3). Since dopamine has been deemed the most important of all neurotransmitters in the neurological expression of pleasure, it is a defect in the gene that carries this chemical that has been primarily blamed for the incidence of this disorder.

The D2 Dopamine-Receptor Gene
The D2 receptor has been determined the producer of the "reward"-producing neurotransmitters, and there are two main variants of the gene that contains this chemical: the A1 allele and the A2 allele.
(http://www.sigmaxi.org/amsci/captions/captions96-03/blum-6.html - link to diagram of gene's variants) (3).

Carriers of the A1 allele are said to be predisposed to reward deficiency syndrome for the simple reason that they have about thirty percent fewer D2 receptors than carriers of the A2 allele.

(http://www.sigmaxi.org/amsci/captions/captions96-03/blum-10.html - link to diagram comparing dopamine

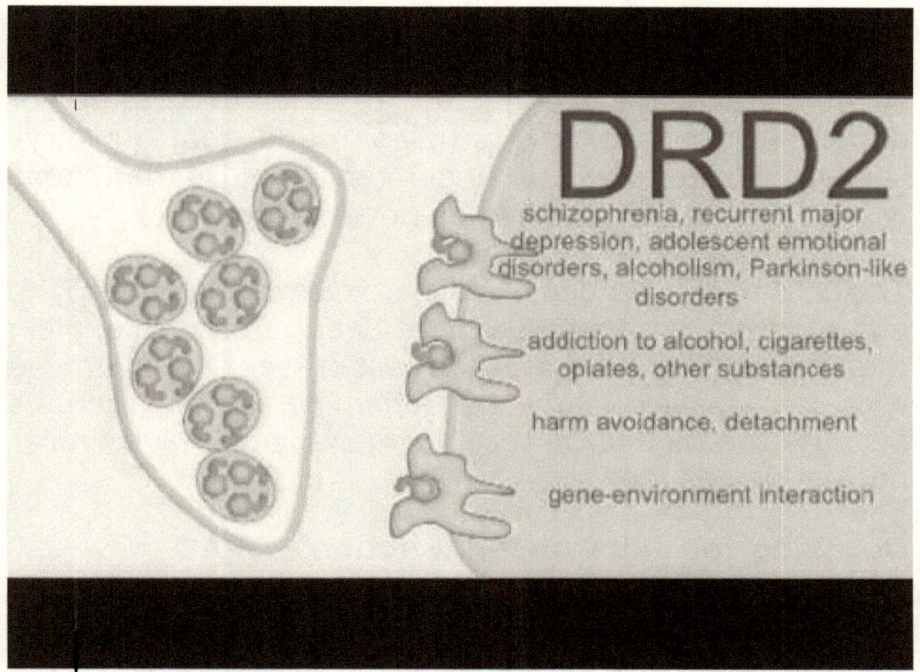

receptor numbers in an A1 allele and an A2 allele) (3). Thus, it is more likely that there are lower levels of dopamine-related activity in the brains of Al-allele carriers than in the brains of A2 carriers. And since dopamine plays a role in reducing stress as well, individuals with the A1 allele may depend on dopamine-releasing substances such as marijuana, alcohol, chocolate, and others to respond to their own stress or cravings.

The D4 Dopamine-Receptor Gene
The dopamine D2 receptor gene is thought to be the most instrumental in determining whether or not an individual will be diagnosed with reward deficiency syndrome or not; however, other genes - such as the D4 receptor gene - are believed to be involved in different expressions of the disorder. For instance, Israeli and National Institute of Mental Health scientists recently found that carriers of

a certain form of the D4 gene are inclined to partake in novelty or sensation-seeking activities.

The objective of their studies was to test Washington University scientist Robert Cloninger's hypothesis that such behavior is connected to the processing of dopamine. Indeed, the studies found that novelty-seekers tended to have a longer version of D4 than those who could not be classified as novelty-seekers.

The latter group tended to be more calm, reflective, loyal, and rigid (3). A reason that has been offered to explain the similarity between these sensation-seekers and those with the A1 allele of the D2 dopamine receptor gene is because the D2 and D4 receptor-genes both have similar nucleotide sequences.

Detoxing for Substance Addiction - QFAC

REWARD DEFICIENCY SYNDROME (RDS) has affected many people's lives either as a child, parent, sibling or spouse. Sadly, one third of the population expresses one form or another of Reward Deficiency Syndrome behavior. In the majority of people, dopamine has been singled out as "the primary neurotransmitter of reward." As a result, one feels "secure, calm, comfortable and satisfied," referred to as the "reward." In fact, a lot of research has shown that a significant amount of human behavior is aimed towards achieving such feelings.

How Can you Recognize Reward Deficiency Syndrome?

* Addictive Behaviors

* Alcoholism

* Polysubstance Abuse

* Obesity

* Impulsive

* ADHD (Attention Deficit Hyperactivity Disorder)

*   Personality Disorder
*   Conduct Disorder
*   Antisocial Personality
*   Aggressive Behavior
*   Pathological Gambling
*   Compulsive Disorders

The relationship between low dopamine levels and addictive behavior is key to helping physicians treat patients in a primary care setting. Physicians nowadays, who treat addiction no longer inflict cold turkey (symptoms of chills and gooseflesh that accompanied opioid and alcohol withdrawal) detox on patients. "Cold Turkey" has proven to be ineffective and inhumane. Addicted patients who were unable to endure withdrawal often returned to drugs to obtain relief. Few made it through the detox process, some even died.

An important fact to keep in mind when thinking about detoxification is that sudden withdrawal - especially from the sedative/hypnotic drugs like alcohol and benzodiazepines - can kill. Proper detoxification process should be done safely and comfortably, as it increases the likelihood that those suffering from addiction problems will seek treatment at an earlier stage of their illness, and will transition from treatment to long-term sobriety with greater confidence. Proper detox makes it much more likely that addicts will seek treatment at an earlier stage of their illness, and will transition from treatment to long-term sobriety with greater confidence.

Excel Treatment Program offers a comprehensive diagnostic drug and alcohol treatment clinic that's dedicated to the growing population of this devastating disease. They have implemented the most effective state of the art technology in the treatment of this disease. Excel Treatment is one out of only five clinics in the

United States that enforces the treatment in genetic and environmental addictions. Excel utilizes diagnostic gene testing when needed to test for alcohol genetic predisposition.

This treatment is currently offered in the state of Colorado and Nevada, and is in the process of the process of negotiating franchises in 5 states. Excel is changing and repairing the biochemistry of the brain by understanding the genetic DNA that at birth contains the gene of addiction. Beat the war on addiction!

Reward deficiency syndrome: Genetic aspects of behavioral disorders by Comings DE, Blum K Department of Medical Genetics, City of Hope Medical Center,Duarte, CA 91010, USA. dcomings@earthlink.net Prog Brain Res 2000; 126:325-41

ABSTRACT
The dopaminergic and opioidergic reward pathways of the brain are critical for survival since they provide the pleasure drives for eating, love and reproduction; these are called 'natural rewards' and involve the release of dopamine in the nucleus accumbens and frontal lobes. However, the same release of dopamine and production of sensations of pleasure can be produced by 'unnatural rewards' such as alcohol, cocaine, methamphetamine, heroin, nicotine, marijuana, and other drugs, and by compulsive activities such as gambling, eating, and sex, and by risk taking behaviors.

Since only a minority of individuals become addicted to these compounds or behaviors, it is reasonable to ask what factors distinguish those who do become addicted from those who do not. It has usually been assumed that these behaviors are entirely voluntary and that environmental factors play the major role; however, since all of these behaviors have a significant genetic component, the presence of one or more variant genes presumably act as risk factors for these behaviors.

Since the primary neurotransmitter of the reward pathway is dopamine, genes for dopamine synthesis, degradation, receptors, and transporters are reasonable candidates. However, serotonin, norepinephrine, GABA, opioid, and cannabinoid neurons all modify dopamine metabolism and dopamine neurons. We have proposed that defects in various combinations of the genes for these neurotransmitters result in a Reward Deficiency Syndrome (RDS) and that such individuals are at risk for abuse of the unnatural rewards. Because of its importance, the gene for the [figure: see text] dopamine D2 receptor was a major candidate gene.

Studies in the past decade have shown that in various subject groups the Taq I A1 allele of the DRD2 gene is associated with alcoholism, drug abuse, smoking, obesity, compulsive gambling, and several personality traits. A range of other dopamine, opioid, cannabinoid, norepinephrine, and related genes have since been added to the list.

Like other behavioral disorders, these are polygenically inherited and each gene accounts for only a small per cent of the variance. Techniques such as the Multivariate Analysis of Associations, which simultaneously examine the contribution of multiple genes, hold promise for understanding the genetic make up of polygenic disorders.

Reward deficiency syndrome: a biogenetic model for the diagnosis and treatment of impulsive, addictive, and compulsive behaviors.

Blum K, Braverman ER, Holder JM, Lubar JF, Monastra VJ, Miller D, Lubar JO, Chen TJ, Comings DE.
Department of Biological Sciences, University of North Texas, Denton, Texas, USA.

The dopaminergic system, and in particular the dopamine D2 receptor, has been implicated in reward mechanisms. The net effect of neurotransmitter interaction at the mesolimbic brain region induces "reward" when dopamine (DA) is released from the neuron at the nucleus accumbens and interacts with a dopamine D2 receptor.

"The reward cascade" involves the release of serotonin, which in turn at the hypothalamus stimulates enkephalin, which in turn inhibits GABA at the substania nigra, which in turn fine tunes the amount of DA released at the nucleus accumbens or "reward site." It is well known that under normal conditions in the reward site DA works to maintain our normal drives. In fact, DA has become to be known as the "pleasure molecule" and/or the "anti-stress molecule."

When DA is released into the synapse, it stimulates a number a DA receptors (D1-D5) which results in increased feelings of well-being and stress reduction. A consensus of the literature suggests that when there is a dysfunction in the brain reward cascade, which could be caused by certain genetic variants (polygenic), especially in the DA system causing a hypodopaminergic trait, the brain of that person requires a DA fix to feel good. This trait leads to multiple drug-seeking behavior. This is so because alcohol, cocaine, heroin, marijuana, nicotine, and glucose all cause activation and neuronal release of brain DA, which could heal the abnormal cravings.

Certainly after ten years of study we could say with confidence that carriers of the DAD2 receptor A1 allele have compromised D2 receptors. Therefore lack of D2 receptors causes individuals to have a high risk for multiple addictive, impulsive and compulsive behavioral propensities, such as severe alcoholism, cocaine, heroin, marijuana and nicotine use, glucose bingeing, pathological gambling, sex addiction, ADHD, Tourette's

Syndrome, autism, chronic violence, Posttraumatic stress disorder, schizoid/avoidant cluster, conduct disorder and antisocial behavior.

In order to explain the breakdown of the reward cascade due to both multiple genes and environmental stimuli (pleiotropism) and resultant aberrant behaviors, Blum united this hypodopaminergic trait under the rubric of a reward deficiency syndrome.

Chapter Eight
Reward Deficiency Syndrome

Scientists postulate that a biological condition known as "reward deficiency syndrome" may predispose up to 88 million individuals in the United States to addiction and/or other psycho-pathological behaviors.

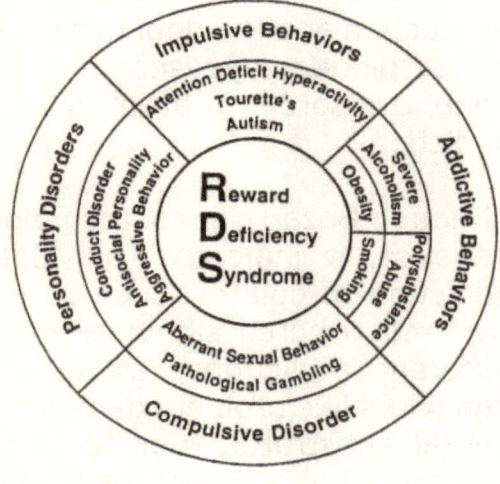

The syndrome is defined by small abnormalities in brain-reward processes involving specific neural pathways. It is suspected in some cases to have a genetic component that may predispose some individuals to addiction-not only to strong stimulants like opiates but to weaker stimulants like alcohol, nicotine, gambling, sex, violence, cannabis and food.

Michael Bozarth, associate professor of psychology, was among a small number of scientists whose research originally suggested an empirical relationship between the neurotransmitter dopamine, which is associated with feelings of pleasure, and certain addictions.

Bozarth, director of the Addiction Research Unit in the Department of Psychology in the College of Arts and Letters, presented an invited lecture on this subject to the First Conference on Reward Deficiency Syndrome: Genetic Antecedents and Clinical Pathways, held Nov. 12-13, 2001 in San Francisco, California USA.

He addressed the relationship between neural-reward mechanisms and normal and pathological behavior, and specifically, the dopamine link as a target for therapeutic intervention in addictive behavior. Those participating in the meeting included many scientists whose studies suggest a relationship between addiction, dopamine production and the dopamine D2 receptor, and scientists whose pioneering research suggests the possibility of a genetic disorder that predisposes tens of millions to addiction.

Although Bozarth's research did not involve the study of genetics, it indicates that dopamine plays a role in addiction to opiates, such as heroin and morphine. His work contributed significantly to the current view that different addictions, as well as psycho-pathological behaviors like problem gambling, may involve a common neural substrate. Prior to this finding, scientists had assumed that different mechanisms were responsible for various substance-abuse disorders.

Bozarth points out that in healthy individuals, normal life activities provoke the release of dopamine, which evokes feelings of pleasure. It is presumed that in some individuals, however, this reward system in brain is not working properly.

"Their brains appear to release less dopamine than might be expected under normal circumstances or the released dopamine has less effect because its receptors in the brain are not functioning properly," Bozarth says. "This may be because of depression or other underlying pathology, some of which are genetically based."

Under most circumstances, he says, such people may be relatively anhedonic-that is, unable to feel pleasure to the same extent as most people. Even people with normal, healthy brains can be easily addicted to drugs like cocaine and heroin, Bozarth says, because such drugs provoke the release of a flood of dopamine, producing pleasure so intense that it often results in a craving that can, in turn, can lead to addiction.

"Some scientists postulate that individuals whose brains do not release dopamine in normal quantities, or do not have properly functioning receptors for dopamine, would be particularly susceptible to addiction," he says.

"This is because when they are introduced to an external stimulant, the feelings of pleasure produced are extremely intense compared to what they normally experience. They are overwhelmed by a craving so profound that the pursuit of the stimulant begins to take over their lives. They seem to lose control over their own behavior. The brain actually changes.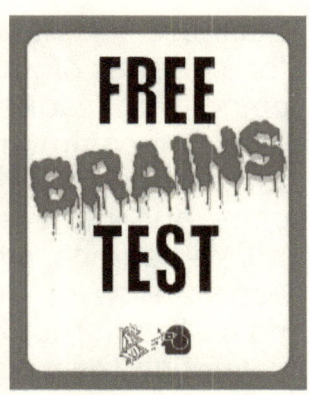

"It is further postulated," he says, "that such individuals are vulnerable not just to extremely addictive drugs like heroin or cocaine, which as I said, can addict even normal brains, but to weaker stimulants as well —alcohol, nicotine, gambling, sex, food. In this case, too, the pleasure they receive from exposure to these stimulants so far exceeds what they normally feel that a craving is set up even to the lesser stimulants."

Bozarth emphasizes, however, that while some such addictions may indeed be produced by dopamine deprivation, "it is certainly the case that not all substance-abuse disorders are caused by a common action on a single brain system.

"What has spawned a new way of looking at addiction," he says, "is the fact that many of the potent motivational, and hence addictive, properties of different substances seem to involve a common neurochemical action. The (San Francisco) conference will address new findings about the relationship between neurotransmitters, their receptors in the brain and addictive action."

The conference theme: C.A.N. - CONTROLLING ADDICTION NATURALLY ADDICTION - HOW BIG A PROBLEM?

There are individual, family, community, national and global scenes of immense distress and pain in living and coping with addictive and compulsive behaviors, that costs our communities billions of dollars. Any addict's journey takes them firstly, in pursuit of another time and space, and into a growing loss of trust by all sides, daily and sometimes even hourly disorder, depression and despair. How can we improve our understanding, care and addiction recovery approaches to ensure that we are all working towards our greatest human potential?

Chapter Nine
Diagnosing the Problem

The Braverman Nature self-assessment instrument included hereafter is provided as a means of determining brain-based influences upon mental health and functionality. The scores are to be 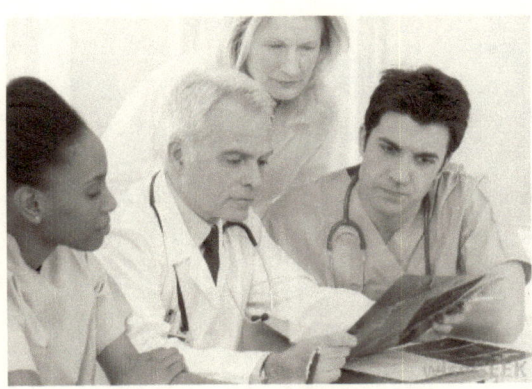 interpreted by your professional team of health care providers. It is not intended as a substitute for medical treatment. While blood tests are considered the most accurate means of assessing the levels of neurotransmitters, this assessment instrument has been found to correlate closely with the results of blood tests.

Instructions
Answer each question by choosing either True or False. Answer the questions in terms of how you feel most of the time, not just at the present moment. For example, if you had a bad night's sleep and feel more tired today than normal, answer the questions pertaining to your energy levels based on how you feel on an average day.

Print out the Braverman Nature Assessment beginning on the following page and complete it.
Check only those statements where your response is TRUE. Add up all of the statements checked, giving yourself one point for each statement checked. Park your score at the bottom of each group of questions. (there are 8 groups or parts). Parts 1-A through 4-A reveal your dominant nature while Parts B-1 through B-4 reveal your present deficiency of the essential reward hormones.

At the end of the assessment there is a place for you to record the number of true statements from each group.

PART 1: Determining Your Dominant Nature

Part 1-A

Memory and Attention

1 ___ I find it easy to process my thoughts.
2. ___ I concentrate effectively.
3. ___ I am a deep thinker.
4. ___ I am a quick thinker.
5. ___I become distracted because I do so many tasks at once.
6. ___I enjoy intense debate.
7. ___I have a good imagination.
8. ___I tend to criticize and analyze my thoughts.

Physical

9. ___ I have a lot of energy most of the time.
10. ___My blood pressure is often elevated.
11. ___Sometimes in my life I have had episodes of extreme energy.
12. ___ 1 have insomnia.
13 ___ I find exercising invigorating.
14.___ I don't ordinarily need coffee to jump start me in the morning.
15. ___My veins are visible and tend to ' out of my skin'
16. ___I tend to have a high body temperature.
17. ___I eat my lunch while I'm working.
18. ___I engage in sexual intercourse any chance I can get.
19. ___I have a temper.
20. ___I eat only to re-energize my body.
21. ___I love action movies.
22. ___Exercising makes me feel powerful.

Personality

23. ___I am a very domineering individual.
24. ___I sometimes don' notice my feelings.
25. ___I have trouble sometimes listening to others because my own ideas dominate.
26. ___I have been in many physical altercations.
27. ___I tend to be future oriented.
28.___ 1 am sometimes speculative.

29. ___Most people view me as thinking oriented.
30. ___I daydream and often fantasize.
31. ___1 like to read nonfiction and factual history.
32. ___1 admire ingenuity.
33. ___1 can be slow in identifying how people can cause trouble.
34. ___I don't usually get tricked by people who say they need my help.
35. ___Most people view me as innovative.
36. ___People have thought I have had some strange ideas, but I can always explain the basis for them rationally.
37. ___I am often agitated or irritated.
38. ___Little things make me anxious or upset.
39. ___I have fantasies of unlimited power.
40. ___ I love spending money.
41. ___I dominate others in my relationships.
42. ___I am very hard on myself.
43. ___I react aggressively to criticism, often becoming defensive in front of others.

Character
44. ___ Some individuals view me as tough-minded.
45. ___Most people view me as achievement oriented.
46. ___Some people say that I am irrational.
47. ___1 will do anything to reach a goal.
48. ___I value a religious philosophy.
49. ___Incompetence makes me angry.
50. ___I have high standards for myself and for others.

___ **Total # of True responses in Part 1-A:**

Part 2-A.
Memory and Attention
1. ___My memory is very strong.
2. ___I am an excellent listener.
3. ___I am good at remembering stories.
4. ___I usually do not forget a face.
5. ___I am very creative.
6. ___I have an excellent attention span and rarely miss a thing.
7. ___I have many good ideas

8. ___I notice everything going on around me.
9. ___I have a good imagination.

Physical
10. ___I tend to have a slow pulse.
11. ___My body has excellent tone.
12. ___I have a great figure/build.
13. ___I have low cholesterol.
14. ___When I eat, I love to experience the aromas and the beauty of food.
15. ___I love yoga and stretching my muscles.
16. ___During sex I am very sensual.
17. ___I have had an eating disorder at some point in my life.
18. ___I have tried many alternative remedies.

Personality
19. ___I am a perpetual romantic.
20. ___I am in touch with my feelings.
21. ___I tend to make decisions based on hunches.
22. ___I like to speculate.
23. ___Some people say I have my head in the clouds.
24. ___I love reading fiction.
25. ___I have a rich fantasy life.
26. ___I am creative when solving people problems.
27. ___I am very expressive; I like to talk about what's bothering me.
28. ___I am buoyant.
29. ___I believe that it is possible to have a mystical experience.
30. ___I believe in being a soul mate.
31. ___Sometimes the mystical can excite me.
32. ___I tend to overreact to my body.
33. ___I find it easy to change; I am not set in my ways.
34. ___I am deeply in touch with my emotions.
35. ___I tend to love someone one minute and hate him or her the next.
36. ___I am flirtatious.
37. ___I don't mind spending money if it benefits my relationships.
38. ___I tend to fantasize when I'm having sex.
39. ___My relationships tend to be filled with romance.

40. ___ I love watching romantic movies.
41. ___ I take risks in my love life.

Character
42. ___ I foresee a better future.
43. ___ I am inspired to help other people.
44. ___ I believe that all things are possible particularly for those who are devoted.
45. ___ I am good at creating harmony between people.
46. ___ Charity and altruism come from the heart, and I have plenty of both.
47. ___ I am thought of by others as having vision.
48. ___ My thoughts on religion often change.
49. ___ I am an idealist, but not a perfectionist.
50. ___ I'm happy with someone who just treats me right.

___ **Total # of True responses in Part 2-A**

Part 3-A.
Memory and Attention
1. ___ I have a stable attention span and can follow other people's logic.
2. ___ I enjoy reading people more than books.
3. ___ I retain most of what I hear.
4. ___ I can remember facts people tell me.
5. ___ I learn from my experiences.
6. ___ I am good at remembering names.
7. ___ I can focus very well on tasks and people's stories.

Physical
8. ___ I find it easy to relax.
9. ___ I am a calm person.
10. ___ I find it easy to fall asleep at night.
11. ___ I tend to have high physical endurance.
12. ___ I have low blood pressure.
13. ___ I do not have a family history of stroke.
14. ___ When it comes to sex, I am not very experimental.
15. ___ 1 have little muscle tension.
16. ___ Caffeine has little effect on me.

17. ___I take my time eating my meals.
18. ___I sleep well.
19. ___I don' have many harmful food cravings such as sugar.
20. ___Exercising is a regimented habit for me.

Personality
21. ___I am not very adventurous.
22. ___I do not have a temper.
23. ___I have a lot of patience.
24. ___I don't enjoy philosophy.
25. ___I love watching sitcoms about real families.
26. ___I dislike movies about other worlds or universes.
27. ___I am not a risk-taker.
28. ___I keep past experiences in mind before I make decisions.
29. ___I am a realistic person.
30. ___I believe in closure.
31. ___I like facts and details.
32. ___When I make a decision, it's permanent.
33. ___I like to plan my day, week, month, etc.
34. ___I collect things.
35. ___I am a little sad.
36. ___I'm afraid of confrontations and altercations.
37. ___I save up a lot of money in the event of a crisis.
38. ___I tend to create strong, lasting bonds with others.
39. ___I am a stable pillar in people's lives.

Character
40. ___I believe in early to bed early to rise.
41. ___I believe in meeting deadlines.
42. ___I try to please others the best I can.
43. ___I am a perfectionist.
44. ___I am good at maintaining long lasting relationships.
45. ___I pay attention to where my money goes.
46. ___I believe that the world would be more peaceful if people would improve their morals.
47. ___I am very loyal, and devoted to my loved ones.
48. ___I have high ethical standards that I live by.
49. ___I pay close attention to laws, principles and policies.
50. ___I believe in participating in service for the community.

Part 4-A.
Memory and Attention
1. ___I can easily concentrate on manual labor tasks.
2. ___I have a good visual memory.
3. ___I am very perceptive.
4. ___I am an impulsive thinker.
5. ___I live in the ' and now'
6. ___I tend to say " me the bottom line."
7. ___I am a slow book learner but I learn from experience.
8. ___I need to experience something or work at is "hands on" in order to understand it.

Physical
9. ___I sleep too much.
10. ___When it comes to sex, I am very experimental.
11. ___I have low blood pressure.
12. ___I am very action-oriented.
13. ___I am very handy around the house.
14. ___I am very active outdoors.
15. ___1 engage in daring activity such as skydiving, motorcycle riding, etc.
16. ___I can solve problems spontaneously.
17. ___I rarely have carbohydrate cravings.
18. ___I usually grab a quick meal on the run.
19. ___I'm not very consistent with my exercise routine; I may exercise daily for three weeks and then forget all about it for a month.

Personality
20. ___1 live life in the immediate moment.
21. ___I like to perform/entertain in public.
22. ___I tend to gather facts in an unorganized manner.
23. ___I am very flexible.
24. ___I am a great negotiator.
25. ___I often just like to "eat, drink, and be merry."
26. ___I am dramatic.
27. ___I am very artistic.

28. ___I am a good craftsman.
29. ___I'm a risk-taker when it comes to sports.
30. ___I believe in psychics.
31. ___1 can easily take advantage of others.
32. ___I am cynical of other' philosophies.
33. ___I like to have fun.
34. ___My favorite type of movies are horror flicks.
35. ___I am fascinated with weapons.
36. ___I rarely stick to a plan or agenda.
37. ___I have trouble remaining faithful.
38. ___I am easily able to separate and move on when relationships with loved ones end.
39. ___I don't pay much attention to how I spend my money.
40. ___I have many frivolous relationships.

Character
41. ___I always keep my options open in case something better comes up.
42. ___I don' like working hard for long periods of time.
43. ___I believe things should have a function and purpose.
44. ___I am optimistic.
45. ___I live in the moment.
46. ___I pray only when I'm in need of spiritual support.
47. ___I don't have particularly high morals and ethical values.
48. ___I do what I want, when I want to.
49. ___I don't care about being perfect, I just live my life.
50. ___Savings are for suckers.

___Total # of True responses in Part 4-!:

Part A Results
___ 1A. Total "" Responses: Dopamine Nature
___ 2A. Total "" Responses: Acetylcholine Nature
___ 3A. Total "" Responses: GABA Nature
___ 4A. Total "" Responses: Serotonin Nature

Scoring Your Braverman Nature Assessment
The category with the most true responses will identify your dominant nature. A classically dominant nature is typically a score

of 35 and above in any one category, which suggests a less than balanced life. When any other nature(s) is 10-15 points lower, i.e.. a score reading 40 Dopamine, 33 Acetylcholine, 25 GABA, and 17 Serotonin, it would appear that GABA and Serotonin are life long relative deficiencies needing balance even in times of good health.

Part Two: Defining Your Presenting Deficiencies

Instructions: Check each statement that is true. At the end of each group, record the total number of True statements in the space provided. The second assessment will determine if you are deficient in any of the four biochemicals, including the one that governs your nature. Many of the questions relate to symptoms you might be experiencing. Answer the questions in terms of how you feel right now: it doesn't matter how long you've been experiencing these symptoms, even if they occurred today for the first time. You will refer to this sheet in subsequent chapters to classify physical symptoms and select treatment alternatives that address your nature and restore your natural well-being.

Part I-B.
Memory and Attention

1. ___I have trouble paying consistent attention and concentrating.
2. ___I need caffeine to wake up.
3. ___I cannot think quickly enough.
4. ___I do not have a good attention span.
5. ___I have trouble getting through a task even when it is interesting to me.
6. ___I am slow in learning new ideas.

Physical

7. ___I crave sugar.
8. ___I have decreased libido.
9. ___I sleep too much.
10. ___I have a history of alcohol or addiction.
11. ___I have recently felt worn out for no apparent reason.
12. ___I sometimes experience total exhaustion without even exerting myself.

13. ___I have always battled weight problems.
14. ___I have little motivation for sexual experiences.
15. ___I have trouble getting out of bed in the morning.
16. ___I have had a craving for cocaine, amphetamines, or Ecstasy.

Personality
17. ___1 feel fine just following others.
18. ___People seem to take advantage of me.
19. ___I am feeling very down or depressed.
20. ___People have told me I am too mellow.
21. ___1 have little urgency.
22. ___I let people criticize me.
23. ___I always look to others to lead me.

Character
24. ___I have lost my reasoning skills.
25. ___I can' make good decisions.

___**Total # of True responses in Part 1-B:**

Part 2-B.
Memory and Attention
1. ___I lack imagination.
2. ___I have difficulty remembering names when I first meet people.
3. ___I have noticed my memory ability is decreasing.
4. ___My significant other tells me I don' have romantic thoughts.
5. ___I can't remember my friends birthdays.
6. ___I have lost some of my creativity.

Physical
7. ___I have insomnia.
8. ___I have lost muscle tone.
9. ___I don't exercise any more.
10. ___I crave fatty foods.
11. ___I have experimented with hallucinogenics, LSD, or other illicit drugs.
12. ___I feel like my body is falling apart.

13. ___ I can't breathe easily.

Personality
14. ___ I don' feel joy very often.
15. ___ I feel despair.
16. ___ I protect myself from being hurt by others by never telling much about myself.
17. ___ I find it more comfortable to do things alone rather than in a large group.
18. ___ Other people get angrier about bothersome things than I do.
19. ___ I give in easily and tend to be submissive.
20. ___ I rarely feel passionate about anything.
21. ___ I like routine.

Character
22. ___ I don' care about anyone' stories but mine.
23. ___ I don' pay attention to people' feelings.
24. ___ I don' feel buoyant.
25. ___ I'm obsessed with my deficiencies.

___ **Total # of True responses in Part 2-B:**

Part 3-B.
Memory and Attention
1. ___ I find it difficult to concentrate because I'm nervous and jumpy.
2. ___ I can't remember phone numbers.
3. ___ I have trouble finding the ' word'
4. ___ I have trouble remembering things when I am put on the spot.
5. ___ I know I am intelligent, but it is hard to show others.
6. ___ My ability to focus comes and goes.
7. ___ When I read, I find I have to go back over the same paragraph a few times to absorb the information.
8. ___ I am a quick thinker, but can' always say what I mean.

Physical
9. ___ I feel shaky.

10. ___I sometimes tremble.
11. ___I have frequent backaches and/or headaches.
12. ___I tend to have shortness of breath.
13. ___1 tend to have heart palpitations.
14. ___I tend to have cold hands.
15. ___I sometimes sweat too much.
16. ___I am sometimes dizzy.
17. ___I often have muscle tension.
18. ___I tend to get butterflies in my stomach.
19. ___I crave bitter foods.
20. ___I am often nervous.
21. ___I like yoga because it helps me to relax.
22. ___1 often feel fatigued even when I have had a good night's sleep.
23. ___I overeat.

Personality
24. ___I have mood swings.
25. ___I enjoy doing many things at one time, but I find it difficult to decide what to do first.
26. ___1 tend to do things just because I think they' be fun.
27. ___When things are dull, I always try to introduce some excitement.
28. ___I tend to be fickle, changing my mood and thoughts frequently.
29. ___I tend to get overly excited about things.
30. ___My impulses tend to get me into a lot of trouble.
31. ___I tend to be theatrical and draw attention to myself.
32. ___I speak my mind no matter what the reaction of others may be.
33. ___1 sometimes have fits of rage and then feel terrible guilty.
34. ___I often tell lies to get out of trouble.
35. ___1 have always had less interest than the average person in sex.

Character
36. ___I don' play by the rules anymore.
37. ___I have lost many friends.
38. ___I can' sustain romantic relationships.

39. ___ 1 consider the law arbitrary without reason.
40. ___I consider rules that I use to follow hopeless.

___**Total # of True responses in Part 3-B:**

Part 4-B.
Memory and Attention
1. ___I am not very perceptive.
2. ___I can't remember things that I have seen in the past.
3. ___I have a slow reaction time.
4. ___I have a poor sense of direction.

Physical
5. ___I have night sweats.
6. ___I have insomnia.
7. ___I tend to sleep in many different positions in order to feel comfortable.
8. ___I always awake early in the morning.
9. ___I can' relax.
10. ___1 wake up at least two times per night.
11. ___It is difficult for me to fall back asleep when I am awakened.
12. ___1 crave salt.
13. ___I have less energy to exercise.
14. ___I am sad.

Personality
15. ___I have chronic anxiety.
16. ___I am easily irritated.
17. ___I have thoughts of self-destruction.
18. ___I have had suicidal thoughts in my life.
19. ___I tend to dwell on ideas too much.
20. ___I am sometimes too structured that I become inflexible.
21. ___My imagination takes over.
22. ___Fear grips me.

Character
23. ___I can' stop thinking about the meaning of life.
24. ___I no longer want to take risks.

25. ___The lack of meaning in my life is painful to me.

___**Total # of True responses in Part 4-B:**

Assessment Results
    Part A   **Part B**
1-A. _____   1-B _____   Dopamine Deficiency
2-A. _____   2-B _____   Acetylcholine Deficiency
3-A. _____   3-B _____   GABA Deficiency
4-A. _____   4-B _____   Serotonin Deficiency

Remember, your scores on Part A represent your dominant nature. Each of the reward hormones predisposes an individual to manifest certain specific character traits.

Dopamine determines how much one is governed by their sense of pleasure – how joyful they tend to be.

Acetylcholine determines how much one is governed by their intellectual energies – their thought processes.

GABA determines whether one tends to be relaxed and easy going or anxious and somewhat uptight.

Serotonin determines one's ability or inability to control their anger, how well they sleep and whether or not they are predisposed to depression.

Should any of your scores be ten or more points less then the average of the others, it means you likely have a chronic deficiency of that hormone. And, should any one of your scores be ten or more points higher than the average of the others, it suggests that you may have an elevated level of that particular reward hormone. Chronic deficiencies or above average levels of any of the reward hormones can predispose a person for certain physical, psychological and/or spiritual disorders or diseases. Any such scores should be discussed with your therapist.

Your scores on Part B represent your presenting state of being – identifying any hormonal deficiencies you may have. A deficiency in any of the reward hormones may predispose a person to specific disorders and/or diseases.

Look at your highest number. This represents your most deficient hormonal nature, the one most likely to lead to illness. If your most deficient nature is the same as your most dominant nature, you'll most likely experience the effects of this deficit sooner than you might otherwise. And if your greatest deficiency on Part B is the same as a chronic deficiency on Part A, it will have a much more pronounced effect.

Look at each of the four reward hormones, or neurotransmitters. If for any hormone you scored 0 to3 on part B that would mean you are in the normal range. Even if your score is a 3 you likely would be experiencing no ill effects.

A score of 4 to 6 would represent a mild deficiency of that hormone. If you scored this on one of more of the neurotransmitters you may experience a mild lack of your sense of well-being, particularly when under stress.

A score of 7 to 9 would represent a moderate deficiency. If you scored this you will no doubt be aware of this deficiency but find that it is not particularly troublesome, except when under stress.

A score of 10 to 12 represents a major deficiency of the hormone or hormones with this score. At this level, you will experience mood disorders and when under stress may exhibit symptoms of personality disorders associated with the particular deficiency.

A score of 13 to 15 represents a profound deficiency of the hormone of hormones with this score. At this level, you will exhibit the symptoms of the personality disorders associated with a deficiency of that hormone, and when under stress will experience one or more of the physical symptoms.

A score of more than 15 on any hormone suggests that you should seek out medical attention as quickly as possible. Deficiencies of this level will result in serious, sometimes life-threatening physiological problems as well as serious mood and personality disorders.

Minor deficits are the early warning signs of health problems. If ignored, they will eventually lead to more serious deficiencies, ultimately affecting your dominant nature, even though they occur in another nature.

Psychosocial Assessment
After administering the Braverman Nature Assessment, if the results indicate that there are deficiencies of more than one neurotransmitter, you will want to conduct a thorough psychosocial assessment interview. There are four things that predispose an individual for RDS:

1] Having a genetic predisposition for addiction - based on having a parent, grandparent, aunt, uncle or sibling who has, or had an addiction to one or more substances or activities such as gambling, pornography, etc.

2] Having suffered a traumatic brain or spinal cord injury, or having experienced one or more periods of unconsciousness, including anesthesia induced unconsciousness for surgery, and any coma including medically induced coma.

3] Having suffered emotional trauma of a profound nature or less severe over a prolonged period of time – particularly during one's developmental years from birth to sixteen.

4] Having a history of personally abusing toxic substances or engaging in addictive activities.

Any one of these suggests the possibility that the person may suffer from RDS while if two of these have occurred in one's life, there is a high probability that the individual suffers from RDS. If three or all four of these things have occurred in one's life, there is a high degree of certainty that the individual suffers from RDS. From a thorough psychosocial assessment interview you will be able to rule in or rule out whether the individual suffers from Reward Deficiency Syndrome [RDS]

Having determined whether one has RDS is only part of the diagnostic process; the other being to determine the severity thereof. This is accomplished by the results of the Braverman Nature Assessment. The greater the level of neurotransmitter deficiencies, the greater the severity of RDS.

To better understand the effects of a hormonal deficiency or a hormone level that is higher than normal level, please refer back to the chapter on "The Biological Connection."

Chapter Ten
Treating RDS

As you have discovered, diagnosing RDS is relatively simple. However, if there is any question about the deficiency levels of the essential reward hormones, or neurotransmitters, this can be verified by other diagnostic procedures such as hair analysis and saliva analysis.

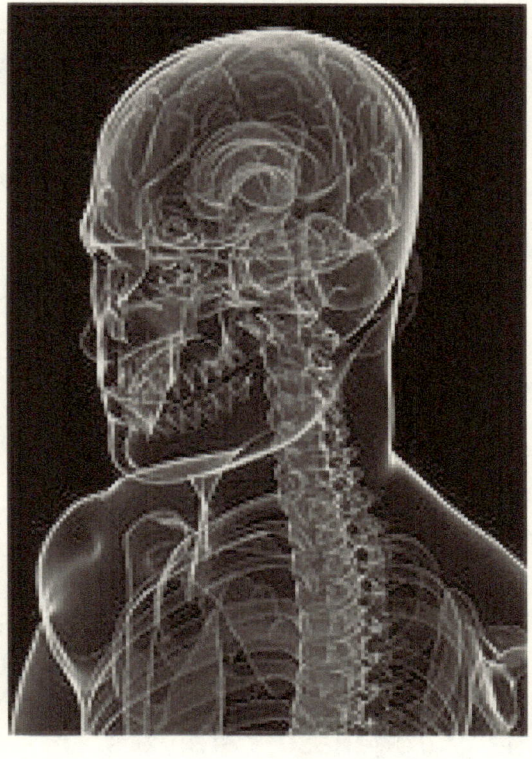

Treating RDS is even less complicated than diagnosing it. For each of the essential reward hormones there is a chemical precursor – an enzyme or Amino Acid. These specific Amino Acids, together with the appropriate vitamin and mineral co-factors will enable the body to begin the process of generating more of these neurotransmitters to restore the appropriate balance.

The most common neurotransmitter imbalances identified in RDS and targeted by the pharmaceutical and neutraceutical industries are Dopamine, GABA, Glutamate, Norepinephrine, and Serotonin. It is well understood that these neurotransmitters are synthesized from specific amino acids obtained from protein in the diet.

All amino acids are derived from intermediates in glycolysis, the citric acid cycle, or the pentose phosphate pathway. Nitrogen enters these pathways by way of glutamate and glutamine. Some pathways are quite simple, others are more complicated. Ten of the amino acids are only one or a few enzymatic steps removed from their precursors. The pathways for others, such as the aromatic amino acids, are much more complex.

Different organisms vary greatly in their ability to synthesize the 20 amino acids. Whereas most bacteria and plants can synthesize all 20 Amino Acids, mammals can synthesize only twelve of them.

Those that are synthesized in mammals are generally those with fairly simple pathways. These are called the nonessential amino acids to denote the fact that they are not needed in the diet. The remainder – the essential amino acids – can only be obtained from food.

Amino acids that must be obtained from the diet are called essential amino acids. Nonessential amino acids are produced in the body. The pathways for the synthesis of nonessential amino acids are quite simple. Glutamate dehydrogenase catalyzes the reductive amination of a-ketoglutarate to glutamate. A transamination reaction takes place in the synthesis of most amino acids. At this step, the chirality of the amino acid is established. Alanine and aspartate are synthesized by the transamination of pyruvate and oxaloacetate, respectively. Glutamine is synthesized from NH4+ and glutamate, and asparagine is synthesized similarly.

Proline and arginine are derived from glutamate. Serine, formed from 3-phosphoglycerate, is the precursor of glycine and cysteine. Tyrosine is synthesized by the hydroxylation of phenylalanine, an essential amino acid.

The pathways for the biosynthesis of essential amino acids are much more complex than those for the nonessential ones. Activated Tetrahydrofolate, a carrier of one-carbon units, plays an important role in the metabolism of amino acids and nucleotides. This coenzyme carries one-carbon units at three oxidation states, which are interconvertible: most reduced—methyl; intermediatemethylene; and most oxidized—formyl, formimino, and methenyl. The major donor of activated methyl groups is S-adenosylmethionine, which is synthesized by the transfer of an adenosyl group from ATP to the sulfur atom of methionine.

S-Adenosylhomocysteine is formed when the activated methyl group is transferred to an acceptor. It is hydrolyzed to adenosine and homocysteine, the latter of which is then methylated to methionine to complete the activated methyl cycle. Cortisol inhibits protein synthesis.

A thorough understanding of the synthesis of Amino Acids requires a comprehensive understanding of biochemistry. Here we will limit the description of this synthesis to the immediate precursors of the essential reward hormones involved in RDS.

Dopamine ~ Dopamine is synthesized in a restricted set of cell types, mainly neurons and cells in the medulla of the adrenal glands. The primary and minor metabolic pathways respectively are:

Primary: L-Phenylalanine   L-Tyrosine   L-DOPA Dopamine

Minor: L-Phenylalanine   L-Tyrosine   p-Tyramine Dopamine

Minor: L-Phenylalanine   m-Tyrosine   m-Tyramine Dopamine

The direct precursor of dopamine, L-DOPA, can be synthesized indirectly from the essential amino acid phenylalanine or directly from the non-essential amino acid tyrosine. These amino acids are found in nearly every protein and are readily available in food, with tyrosine being the most common. Although dopamine is also found in many types of food, it is incapable of crossing the blood–brain barrier that surrounds and protects the brain. It must therefore be synthesized inside the brain to perform its neuronal activity.

L-Phenylalanine is the precursor that is converted into L-tyrosine by the enzyme phenylalanine hydroxylase, with molecular oxygen (O_2) and tetrahydrobiopterin as cofactors. L-Tyrosine is converted into L-DOPA by the enzyme tyrosine hydroxylase, with tetrahydrobiopterin, O_2, and iron (Fe^{2+}) as cofactors. L-DOPA is converted into dopamine by the enzyme aromatic L-amino acid decarboxylase (also known as DOPA decarboxylase), with pyridoxal phosphate as the cofactor.

The most readily available precursor for Dopamine is the Amino Acid L-Tyrosine. However the organic synthesis of L-Tyrosine can be potentated by the addition of its precursor DL-Phenylalanine. DL-Phenylalanine should not be used by anyone with hypertension.

Acetylcholine ~ is an organic chemical that functions in the brain and body of many types of animals, including humans, as a neurotransmitter—a chemical released by nerve cells to send signals to other cells. Its name is derived from its chemical structure: it is an ester of acetic acid and choline. Parts in the body that use or are affected by acetylcholine are referred to as cholinergic. Substances that interfere with acetylcholine activity are called anticholinergics.

Acetylcholine is the neurotransmitter used at the neuromuscular junction – in other words, it is the chemical that motor neurons of the nervous system release in order to activate muscles. This property means that drugs that affect cholinergic systems can have very dangerous effects ranging from paralysis to convulsions.

Acetylcholine is also used as a neurotransmitter in the autonomic nervous system, both as an internal transmitter for the sympathetic nervous system and as the final product released by the parasympathetic nervous system.

Inside the brain, acetylcholine functions as a neuromodulator – a chemical that alters the way other brain structures process information rather than a chemical used to transmit information from point to point. The brain contains a number of cholinergic areas, each with distinct functions. They play an important role in arousal, attention, and motivation.

Acetylcholine is the substance the nervous system uses to activate skeletal muscles, a kind of striated muscle. These are the muscles used for all types of voluntary movement, in contrast to smooth muscle tissue, which is involved in a range of involuntary activities such as movement of food through the gastrointestinal tract and constriction of blood vessels. Skeletal muscles are directly controlled by motor neurons located in the spinal cord or, in a few cases, the brainstem. These motor neurons send their axons through motor nerves, from which they emerge to connect to muscle fibers at a special type of synapse called the neuromuscular junction.

The most readily available precursor supplement for Acetylcholine is SAMe – S-Adenosyl methionine – a common cosubstrate involved in methyl group transfers, transsulfuration, and aminopropylation. Although these anabolic reactions occur throughout the body, most SAM-e is produced and consumed in the liver.

SAMe is a molecule that is formed naturally in the body. It can also be made in the laboratory. SAMe is involved in the formation, activation, or breakdown of other chemicals in the body, including hormones, proteins, phospholipids, and certain drugs.

SAMe has been available as a dietary supplement in the US since 1999, but it has been used as a prescription drug in Italy since 1979, in Spain since 1985, and in Germany since 1989.

SAMe is often taken by mouth for depression, anxiety, heart disease, fibromyalgia, abdominal pain, osteoarthritis, bursitis, tendonitis, chronic lower back pain, dementia, Alzheimer's disease, slowing the aging process, chronic fatigue syndrome (CFS), improving mental performance, liver disease, and Parkinson's disease. It is also used for attention deficit-hyperactivity disorder (ADHD), multiple sclerosis, spinal cord injury, seizures, migraine headache, lead poisoning, to break down a chemical in the body called bilirubin, or to help with disorders related to the buildup of a chemical called porphyrin or its precursors.

Women often take SAMe by mouth for remediating the severity of premenstrual syndrome (PMS) and a more severe form of PMS called premenstrual dysphoric disorder (PMDD).

SAMe is used intravenously (by IV) for depression, osteoarthritis, AIDS-related nervous system disorders, fibromyalgia, liver disease, cirrhosis, and for a liver disorder that occurs in pregnant women called intrahepatic cholestasis. SAMe is injected as a shot for fibromyalgia, depression, and Alzheimer's disease.

GABA ~ Gamma-aminobutyric acid, a neurotransmitter and the cornerstone of the inhibitory (calming) system in the body; controlling the action of epinephrine, norepinephrine, and dopamine. GABA is the body's own endogenous benzodiazapam, an anti-anxiety drug similar to Xanax or Valium.

Inhibitory neurotransmitters and their receptors reduce excitability in the brains neurons and increase the likelihood that an incoming signal will be terminated. For optimal functioning, the brain must balance the excitatory and inhibitory influences: Excessive excitation can lead to seizures, insomnia, anxiety, and many other clinical conditions, whereas excessive inhibition of neurons can result in incoordination, sedation, and anesthesia.

GABA is the primary inhibitory neurotransmitter in the brain and therefore filters out irrelevant messages (static) by terminating signals from the excitatory neurotransmitters: glutamate, and its positive modulators epinephrine, norepinephrine, and PEA. GABA can be viewed as the "braking system" in the realm of neurotransmitters.

In situations where there is high excitatory neurotransmitter activity, the brain typically responds with an increase in the inhibitory GABA activity as well. In essence this slows down neurotransmission by pressing on the GABA "brakes." Under normal conditions, normal levels of GABA are sufficient to maintain control of the excitatory stimuli. If however, GABA function is impaired (worn brakes) then higher levels (pressing harder on the pedal) of GABA are required.

GABA's high concentration in the hypothalamus suggests it plays a significant role in hypothalamic-pituitary function. The hypothalamus is a region of the posterior section of the brain that is the regulating center for visceral (instinctive) functions such as sleep cycles, body temperature and the activity of the pituitary gland.

The pituitary gland is the master endocrine gland affecting all hormone functions of the body. A recent study indicates that GABA also enhances alpha wave production in the brain to promote relaxation and moderate occasional stress. In the same study, it supported healthy IgA levels, suggesting that it may support immune health during occasional stress. Pyridoxal 5'phosphate is an important cofactor involved in the natural synthesis of GABA, providing synergistic support.

Low GABA levels have been found in the brains of patients with multiple sclerosis, action tremors, tardive dyskinesia, & other disorders of movement. Lower than normal GABA levels have been found in individuals suffering from:

- Anxiety
- Panic attacks
- Depression
- Alcoholism
- Bipolar disorders

GABA Synthesis – GABA is formed through the activity of the enzyme glutamic acid decarboxylase (GAD). GAD catalyzes the formation of GABA from glutamic acid. The synthesis of GABA is linked to the Kreb's cycle. GAD requires vitamin B6 (pyridoxal phosphate) as a cofactor, which can be used to regulate the levels of GABA. Vitamin B6 is a key GABA vitamin.

GABA can be metabolized by a transamination reaction with a-ketoglutarate, catalyzed by GABA-transaminase. Compounds such as the competitive GAD inhibitor allylglycine, inhibit GABA formation and cause convulsions due to the lack of GABA activity.

The importance of GABA is underscored by the frequency in which it is a pharmaceutical target and how many commonly used drugs affect its function e.g. Xanax, Klonapin, Valium, Neurontin.

The GABA receptor is a relatively large molecule and has binding sites not only for GABA but also for many modulatory compounds. Many of these modulatory compounds are useful therapeutic agents. Positive GABA modulators, like the benzodiazepines, do not cause the ion channel to open and an influx of chloride ions to occur on their own. They only enhance the activity of naturally occurring GABA by potentiating its function and therefore have vastly reduced potential for overdose or side effects than receptor agonist compounds, like barbiturates.

While much safer than barbiturates benzodiazepine use frequently leads to dependence and withdrawal syndrome effects. This limits their utility for mild/moderate symptoms as well as for long-term therapy.

GABA Positive Effects:
- May reduce symptoms of alcohol withdrawal.
- May reduce symptoms of anxiety.
- May help some schizophrenics.
- May help to reduce high blood pressure.
- May increase the effect of insulin so is useful for diabetics but not for hypoglycemia.
- May suppress appetite.
- May help with premenstrual symptoms.
- Helpful for some cases of depression.

GABA Side Effects:
GABA has little to no side effects. Some sleepiness has been reported.

Hormone (Neurotransmitter)	Nutritional Supplement	Deficiency Symptoms	Potential Abuse & Addiction	Restored Brain Chemicals	Anticipated Behavioral Change
Dopamine	L-Tyrosine DL-Phenylalanine	Lack of Pleasure Loss of Focus Concentrate Issues Loss of Energy Apathy Anhedonia Depression ADD/ADHD	Caffeine, Speed Cocaine, Marijuana Aspartame Chocolate, Sweets Tobacco, Alcohol Starches	Dopamine Norepinepherine	Restored pleasure Increased energy Improved mental concentration & focus Diminished Craving Anti-depression
Acetylcholine	SAMe	Impaired memory Brain Fog Poor Concentration Inability to focus Depression	Caffeine, Speed, Cocaine, Gambling Pornography Stimulants	Adrenaline Epinepherine	Improved memory Improved focus & Concentration
GABA (Gamma-amino butyric acid)	GABA	Feeling Stressed, Tension, Anxiety. Panic Attacks, Difficulty Relaxing, Paranoia	Valium, Xanax, Benzodiazepam, Clonapine, Marijuana. Sweets, Starches, Alcohol	GABA	Improved serenity, Calmness, Ability to Relax, Reduced Anxiety & Paranoia
Serotonin	L-Tryptophan 5-HTP Hydroxltryptophan	Low self-worth, OCD Behaviors Irritability Sleep Disorders Negativity Cravings in PM Fibromyalgia Heat intolerance Seasonal Affective Disorders	Sweets, Starches, Chocolate, Alcohol, Ecstasy, Tobacco, Marijuana, Inhalants	Serotonin	Reduced Craving Anti-depression Anti-insomnia Appetite Control Improved moods Diminished Anger

Enkephalins Endorphins	DL-Phenylalanine D-Phenylalanine	Pain sensitivity, Emotionally sensitivity, hedonism	Heroin, Methadone, Alcohol, Sweets, Starches, Chocolate Tobacco Marijuana	Enkephalins Endorphins	Anti-depression, Improved energy Improved Focus & Concentration Diminished Pain Increased pleasure
Glutamine	L-Glutamine	Stress, Mood Swings Hypoglycemia	Sweets, Starches Alchhol	Glutamine GABA	Diminished Stress Diminished cravings Mood stability Improved Blood Glucose Levels Imcreased energy

Treating Doses ~ To administer the appropriate doses it is important to understand that virtually all the doses of nutritional supplements printed on the labels are maintenance doses for prophylactic or prevention measures. In addition, these maintenance doses are established for an individual weighing 150 pounds.

In consideration of these factors, one must first correlate the maintenance dose with the individual's weight. For example, if the person weighs only 100 pounds a maintenance dose would be two-thirds of that on the label; conversely, if the individual weighs 300 pounds the maintenance dose will be twice what is printed on the label.

Once this adjustment has been made, the deficiencies evident from the individual's scores on the Braverman Nature Assessment must be applied. Applying these values and determining the appropriate dose is relatively simple. On the following page are typical examples which illustrate how to determine the approximate correct doses using this technique. Utilizing Applied Kinesiology insures greater accuracy, but requires specialized training.

A second approach to enhancing the GABA system includes supplementing with GABAs precursors and potentiators. These include the amino acids Taurine, Glutamine, 5-HTP, and Theanine. These amino acids freely cross the blood brain barrier and are a safe, effective option for patients using or considering prescription medications or large doses of GABA.

Phenibut better known as Beta-phenyl-gamma-aminobutyric acid is derived from the neurotransmitter GABA and is capable of crossing the blood brain barrier. Phenibut is cited as a nootropic (that is, "smart drug") for its ability to improve neurological functions. Check out Kavinace, a GABA supplement that contains Phenibut.

Serotonin ~ Serotonin is a natural chemical in the brain and body that functions as both a neurotransmitter and a hormone. It plays many roles in regulating mood, memory, sleep, digestion and more.

Serotonin is the result of an internal biochemical process which combines 5-Hydroxytryptophan (5-HTP) with a chemical reactor called tryptophan hydroxylase. 5-HTP is itself a by-product of the essential amino acid l-tryptophan. Serotonin is derived from the chemical reaction and used by the body for various important purposes.

Both tryptophan and 5-HTP (5-hydroxytryptophan are naturally occurring precursors of the essential neurotransmitter serotonin. Tryptophan is found in collard and turnip greens, poultry, eggs, milk and bananas. These are nutrient-rich foods and excellent additions to the diet. However, the myth that eating a turkey sandwich or drinking a glass of warm milk will make you sleep better is just a myth.

5-Hydroxytryptophan (5-HTP) is the intermediate metabolite of the essential amino acid L-tryptophan (LT) in the biosynthesis of serotonin. Intestinal absorption of 5-HTP does not require the presence of a transport molecule, and is not affected by the presence of other amino acids; therefore it may be taken with meals without reducing its effectiveness. Unlike LT, 5-HTP cannot be shunted into niacin or protein production.

Therapeutic use of 5-HTP bypasses the conversion of LT into 5-HTP by the enzyme tryptophan hydroxylase, which is the rate-limiting step in the synthesis of serotonin. 5-HTP is well absorbed from an oral dose, with about 70 percent ending up in the bloodstream. It easily crosses the blood-brain barrier and effectively increases central nervous system (CNS) synthesis of serotonin. In the CNS, serotonin levels have been implicated in the regulation of sleep, depression, anxiety, aggression, appetite, temperature, sexual behaviour, and pain sensation.

Therapeutic administration of 5-HTP has been shown to be effective in treating a wide variety of conditions, including depression, fibromyalgia, binge eating associated with obesity, chronic headaches, and insomnia. In its role as a neurotransmitter, serotonin regulates the intensity of synaptic signaling. Serotonin plays various other important roles, affecting both bodily and psychological functioning.

Here's a partial list of what serotonin does in the body:
- Regulation of moods, appetite, digestion, social behaviors, libido, sleep and memory;
- Supporting role in the production of breast milk;
- Used for metabolizing bones;
- Maintains cardiovascular system efficiency;
- Helps to regenerates the liver;
- Necessary for efficient cell division

Treatment Protocols
Amino Acid Treatment for Addictions

The amino acids most commonly used to treat addiction are:

- 5-HTP (regulates serotonin levels in the brain)
- GABA (anti-stress)
- DLPA (fights depression)
- L-Tyrosine (building block for neurotransmitters)
- L-Glutamine (nourishes brain cells)

AMINO ACID NUTRITION THERAPY

An important area of the use of nutrition in recovery and relapse prevention is the addition of appropriate amino acids that serve as the building blocks for powerful chemicals in the brain called neurotransmitters. These neurotransmitters, including epinephrine and norepinephrine, GABA, serotonin and dopamine, are closely tied to addiction behavior.

With the use of various amino acids, brain chemistry can be changed to help normalize and restore deficiencies in the neurotransmitters that spur cravings that can lead to addiction and relapse.

Example No. 1 ~ Susan is a 39 year old female weighing 150 pounds. Based on a detailed psychosocial interview she definitely has RDS. Her Braverman Nature Assessment test results are as follows:

Hormone	Part A	Part B
Dopamine	32	10
Acetlycholine	29	6
GABA	33	22
Serotonin	21	16

From her Part A results we know that Susan's dominant nature is a combination of GABA and Dopamine, with Acetylcholine being close behind. Relying on this we know that Susan is a fun-loving individual who is normally quite relaxed and easy-going, with high intellectual energies. In spite of this, Susan has a chronic deficiency of

Serotonin. This has been manifest throughout Susan's life as Dysthymia - a chronic, low-level depression.

Her scores on Part B Susan's greatest deficiency is in GABA, which is also her dominant nature. This results in her GABA deficiency having a more profound effect than it would otherwise. Likewise, the next highest deficiency is in Serotonin, which Susan already has a chronic deficiency in. Once again, her deficiency in Serotonin will have a greater effect than it otherwise would. This has to be taken into account when determining the appropriate doses.

Next, you need to determine both the amount and frequency of the dose of each Amino Acid precursor. One thing you will need to keep in mind is that the majority of the chosen Precursor for Serotonin should be taken before bedtime, while the precursors for the other hormones should be spread out during the day with the last dose being taken before 4:00 pm since they will otherwise tend to keep a person awake during the night.

If the person does not have hypertension (high blood pressure) the effectiveness of the other precursors can be potentiated by adding DLPA - DL-Phenylalanine.

Now, referring back to the deficiency scores, we convert these as follows:

0 to   3 = 1
4 to   6 = 2
7 to   9 = 3
10 to 12 = 4
13 to 15 = 5
16 +   = 6 or more

Using this, the recommended doses for Susan would be as follows:

Hormone   Supplement   Dose   Frequency

Hormone	Supplement	Dose	AM	Noon	4PM	Bed
Dopamine	L-Tyrosine	500mg	2	1	1	
Acetylcholine	SAMe	200mg	1		1	
GABA	GABA	500mg	2	2	2	2
Serotonin	5-HTP	100 mg	2	1		3

If Susan does not have hypertension you could add

	DLPA	500mg	1		1	

If Susan suffers from insomnia it would be best to use L-Tryptophan instead of 5-HTP since the animal based form is more effective when one suffers from insomnia.

Now that we have Susan's recommended doses established, let's consider another patient named Dan.

Dan is a 51 year old male who weighs 290 pounds. Dan suffers from hypertension and insomnia. Based on this, we will want to use L-tryptophan rather than 5-HTP and not add the DLPA. Now, let's examine his scores and determine the recommended doses.

Dan's Braverman scores are as follows:

Hormone	Part A	Part B
Dopamine	28	6
Acetlycholine	29	15
GABA	26	10
Serotonin	30	9

Based on his Part A scores it is apparent that Dan has a very balanced nature. He has no chronic deficiencies and his scores are considerably less pronounced that Susan's. Nevertheless, his score on the Acetlycholine score is at the top of the profound level and his score on the GABA scale is fairly elevated.

From these scores we know that Dan is experiencing rather significant memory impairment, a rather high level of anxiety and moderate depression. These scores give rise to concern that Dan may be experiencing early onset Alzheimer Disease or Dementia, since anxiety, depression and problems controlling anger are frequently associated with these disorders. Our first recommendation therefore would be to evaluate Dan for these disorders, or if this is not within your area of expertise, to refer him to someone who can evaluate him for these disorders.

Let's assume that you have referred Dan to a competent psychologist who has ruled these disorders out. We can now proceed to evaluate his scores and make recommendations based thereon. Remembering that his maintenance dose is twice that on the printed label, The recommended doses for Dan would be as follows:

Hormone	Supplement	Dose	Frequency			
			AM	Noon	4PM	Bed
Dopamine	L-Tyrosine	500mg	2	1	1	
Acetylcholine	SAMe	400mg	1	1	1	
GABA	GABA	500mg	2	2	2	2
Serotonin	L-Tryptophan	500mg	2	1		3

Some individuals experience loose stools when beginning to take Amino Acids. This can be alleviated by commencing the therapy using one-half or one-third the recommended doses, then increasing the doses after a week.

There are a number of compound formulations for different drugs of abuse. However, we prefer using the specific Amino Acids, creating our own personalized formula. Different substances of abuse, and combinations thereof, tend to create their own specific pattern of neurotransmitter deficiencies. In addition, everyone's body chemistry is unique, so personalization of the recommended doses is, we believe, far preferable.

Applied Kinesiology

We mentioned earlier that relying on a thorough psychosocial assessment and the Braverman Nature Assessment provides very good results, but that there is yet a more precise method for determining the correct doses. This is relying on a technique referred to as applied kinesiology or muscle testing. The rudiments of this are depicted in the graphic below, which is explained more fully on the following pages.

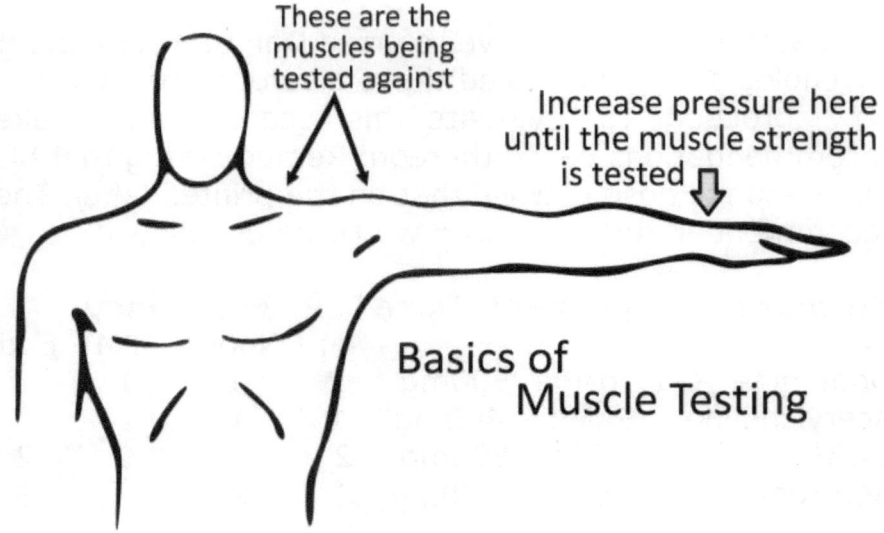

These are the muscles being tested against

Increase pressure here until the muscle strength is tested

Basics of Muscle Testing

Kinesiology ~ also known as biomechanics, is the study of body movement. Applied kinesiology (AK) which is also know as muscle strength testing, is a method of diagnosis and treatment based on the belief that various muscles are linked to particular organs and glands, and that specific muscle weakness can signal distant internal problems such as nerve damage, reduced blood supply, chemical imbalances or other organ or gland problems. Practitioners believe that by correcting this muscle weakness, you help heal the problem in the associated internal organ.

Applied kinesiology can be used to diagnose and treat nervous system problems, nutritional deficiencies or excesses, imbalances in the body's "energy pathways" (known in Traditional Chinese Medicine as meridians). Used in conjunction with the Braverman Nature Assessment, Applied Kinesiology can be used to determine with greater accuracy than relying solely on the Braverman Assessment.

To use this technique you will want to have the person sit in a chair – as shown in the picture at the right – and hold out their dominant hand (the one they write with), palm down. Next, you will want to demonstrate the principles of AK to the person so that they have confidence in what you are doing. To accomplish this, have the person resist you as you take your index and middle finger and begin pressing downward on their wrist until your downward pressure exceeds their ability to resist.

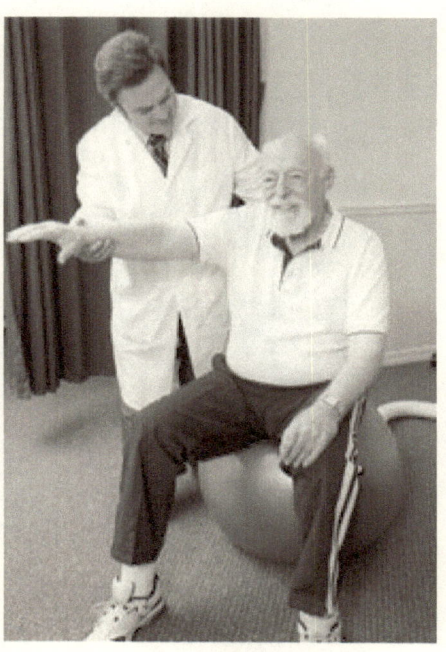

Next, have the person pick up a bottle of water in their other hand, and hold it over their abdomen just below the sternum. Then, while they are holding the water bottle as described, have them resist you as you take your index and middle finger and once again begin slowly applying downward pressure on their wrist until your downward pressure exceeds their ability to resist.

Since water is the universal solvent comprising approximately sixty percent (60%) of the body's weight in women and seventy percent (70%) in men, the body will respond positively and the person's ability to resist you will increase.

After they experience how water can increase their resistance strength, repeat the exercise with the person holding a cup of sugar or a cup of strong coffee below their sternum. These are substances the body normally responds to negatively, noticeably decreasing the person's ability to resist your downward pressure.

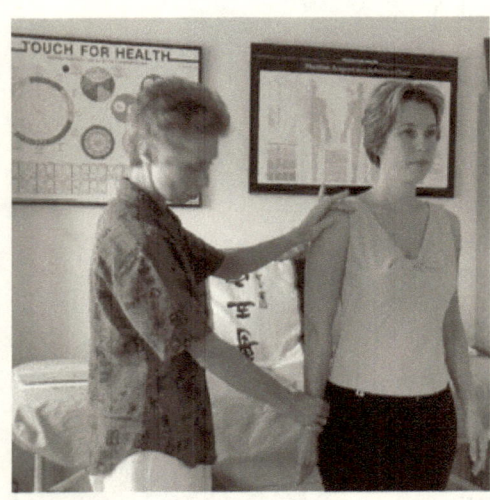

An alternative method shown in the picture left often works better when testing one who is fairly strong. In this method, you will have the person hold their dominant hand to their side, and the water, sugar or coffee in their other hand, as you begin gently pulling their hand away from their body, gradually pulling stronger and stronger until they can no longer keep their arm at their side.

These alternatives will serve as controls demonstrating the efficacy of muscle testing. Once you have completed this control testing, using whichever alternative seems to work best, refer to the results of the person's Braverman Nature Assessment, Part B; and have them hold the bottle containing the supplement that they are most deficient in below their sternum.

Once they feel the positive result, take one of the capsules or caplets from the bottle, and have them hold this in their non-dominant hand just below their sternum as you once again perform the muscle test. Repeat this process, adding another capsule or caplet each time, until their resistance decreases. This is a sign that the dose they are then holding is too much and needs to be decreased.

Repeat this process with each of the supplements that they are deficient in, according to the Braverman Nature Assessment. After you have tested all of the supplements indicated and determined the appropriate doses, apportion them so that they are taken throughout the day. Keep in mind that the majority of the L-Tyrosine should be taken in the morning; SAMe split equally between the morning and afternoon; GABA normally split between morning, noon and afternoon, with them taken also at bedtime by those experiencing panic attacks and/or paranoia.

Approximately sixty percent (60%) of the chosen precursor for Serotonin – either 5-HTP (Hydroxyltryptophan) or L-Tryptophan – should be taken in the evening, just before bedtime, the other forty percent (40%) should be split between the morning and noon. 5-HTP is usually the preferred supplement, however, for individuals suffering from insomnia, the preferred supplement is L-Tyrosine. A 100mg capsule of 5-HTP is equivalent to a 500mg capsule of L-Tryptophan.

If – and only if – the person has no history of hypertension (high blood pressure) the effectiveness of the other Amino Acids can be increased by adding a 500mg capsule of DL- Phanylalanine (DLPA) twice a day, in the morning and afternoon.

Whenever using Amino Acid therapy, it is important that a well-rounded one-a-day vitamin/mineral supplement and additional Vitamin C be taken. These serve as co-factors, speeding and increasing the effectiveness of the synthesis of Amino Acids.

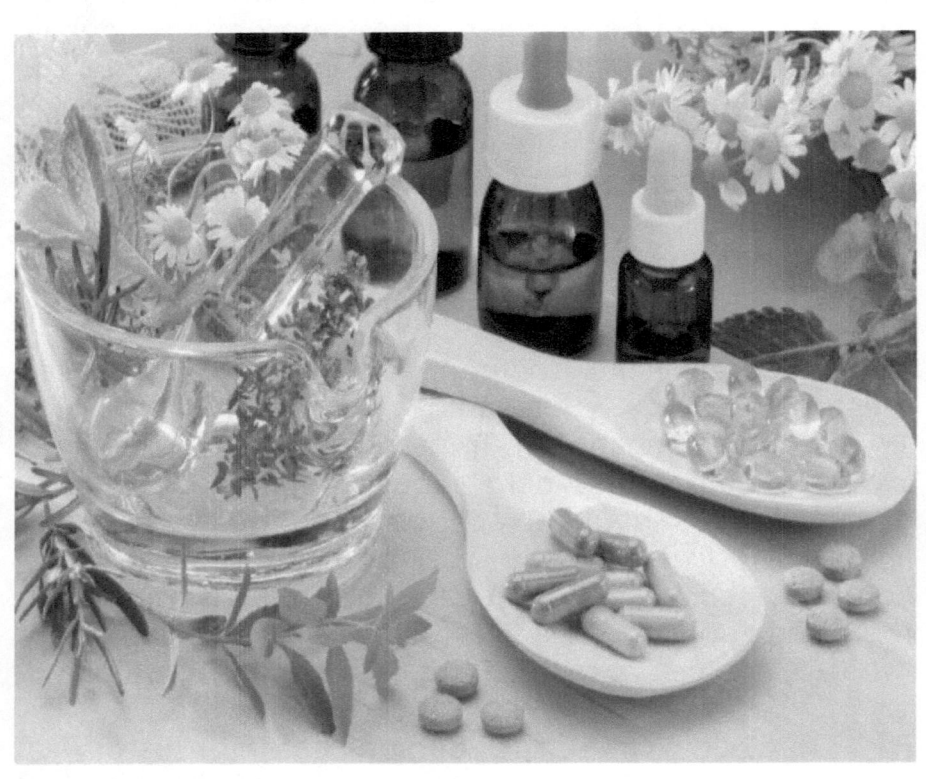

Chapter Eleven
Alternative Treatments

While we believe it is preferable to administer the individual Amino Acids and co-factors determined through Applied Kinesiology and/or the Braverman Nature Assessment, it is worthwhile to mention some of the formulations that have been found to be efficacious in treating various addictions and related disorders.

Alcoholism

According to two excellent books on treating addictions with Amino Acids by Julia Ross – "The Diet Cure" and "The Mood Cure", there is compelling evidence that Amino Acids provide a natural cure for alcoholism.

As Ross points out, the majority of those addicted to alcohol, drugs and food are actually self-medicating in an attempt to feel normal.

Our body depends on proteins to survive. It can manufacture carbohydrates using fats and proteins, and fats, relying on carbohydrates proteins; but it cannot create protein from carbohydrates and fats. Our liver can convert the so-called eight essential proteins into the other twelve, but the essential eight must be ingested.

When we run low on protein, our body and our mind cease to function optimally. When this occurs, our brain signals us to take action to fix the problem. Unfortunately, in our fast-paced world we have learned that carbohydrates (including sugars and alcohol), and certain drugs (both prescription and illicit street drugs) provide a quick "fix". With the regular use of these substances, our body develops a dependency on them, resulting in our body producing fewer and fewer of the essential neurotransmitters.

What does all of this have to do with Amino Acids? A great deal! Our brain relies on proteins, the only source thereof being amino acids. Amino Acids are what our body uses to make all of its mood-enhancing chemicals. If you aren't getting enough protein, or if you have conditioned your brain to interfere with the 'conversion' process, you will start getting cravings. However, this process is reversible: consuming the appropriate amino acid supplements mitigates these cravings. Thus Amino Acids could become a natural cure for alcohol, sugar and other carbohydrate cravings.

When one has an adequate supply of the essential neurotransmitters that govern our moods, we have a sense of well-being; but when our reserves of any of these becomes depleted, we tend to overeat, consume substances that will give us a quick fix, or engage in activities that stimulate the rapid production of the depleted neurotransmitters.

This is why one can become addicted to activities such as gambling, pornography, viewing violent movies, TV and such. They stimulate the production of hormones such as adrenaline, epinepherine, norepinepherine, cortosol, enkephalins, etc. This results in our becoming dependent/addicted to our own internal chemistry.

Correcting this is truly as easy as restoring the reserves of our essential neurotransmitters and insuring that they are in balance. To undertake this, the first neurotransmitter to be addressed is Dopamine or Norepinepherine. The precursor for this is L-Tyrosine – an Amino Acid that works fast, providing additional energy.

The second neurotransmitter one will usually want to address is GABA. Many people abuse alcohol to relax, not realizing that it actually destroys the essential neurotransmitter one must have in order to relax – GABA.

GABA is often called a natural valium (valium is also known as diazepam), used to relieve anxiety as well as side effects associated with alcohol withdrawal. L-Taurine can help relieve tension as well. And, L-theanine will help you reduce stress and relax as well. In other words, adding these three amino acids for your natural cure for alcoholism toolkit!

Alcohol and many other substances are frequently used to self-medicate for emotional pain, but many of these alter the pain threshold over time, making one more sensitive to pain. There are two powerful amino acids used to alleviate emotional pain: L-glutamine and DLPA or DL-Phenylalanine. L-Glutamine is also the second best choice for your body to fuel your brain. Sugar – or glucose – being the primary option. This makes it easy to understand why sugary products, carbohydrates or alcohol, which convert into glucose, easily stop a craving. However, the Amino Acid, L-Glutamine, will reach the brain within just a few minutes.

The last amino acid, L-Tryptophan, is sometimes called "a natural Prozac". When a series of contaminated batches of L-Tryptophan came in from Japan to the U.S. in the late 1980's, the Food and Drug Administration banned it. It was banned for several years, but is again available, and it is a very powerful product. It plays an important role for the synthesis of melatonin and serotonin – hormones that regulate mood and stress response. L-Tryptophan helps support relaxation, sleep, positive mood and immune function. L-Tryptophan is the precursor to Serotonin, a neurotransmitter in the brain, which is deficient in people who have depression. Deficiencies in Serotonin also contribute to alcoholism and many other addictions.

While depleted resources of the essential neurotransmitters lead to chemical dependency and addiction, the supplementation of these has been proven to break the addictive process by addressing the underlying cause of dependency and addiction – an insufficient reserve of these essential neurotransmitters.

Several neutraceutical manufacturers have recognized the benefits of Amino Acid Therapy and are now marketing various formulations thereof. One such product is NeuroRecover™. The manufacturer claims that NeuroRecover™ works for all classes of drugs, including:
- Alcohol
- Antidepressants
- Anxiety drugs (Ativan, Xanax, Klonopin, Valium, etc.)
- Narcotics (pain drugs)
- Heroin and Methadone
- Tobacco
- Marijuana
- Cocaine
- Methamphetamine
- Insomnia drugs
- Stimulants and ADHD drugs

The manufacturer claims that since the formulas are composed entirely of very simple amino acids – the natural building blocks of protein – and a natural enzyme cofactor, they are inherently very safe. They claim that NeuroRecover™ has been found in the majority of cases to bring about major improvement in symptoms of drug and alcohol dependence in a seven- to ten-day period, that otherwise would take months to years to occur (if it would occur at all).

NAD ~ Treatment for Addiction

Another alternative treatment for RDS (formerly addiction) is the infusion of NAD. NAD or Nicatinamide Adenine Dinucleotide is a simple metabolic coenzyme of Niacin. Niacin is a B Vitamin that is involved in enegry production in every mitochondria of your body. It has been used since the early 1930's to help people detox off of alcohol, opiates, stimulants and tranquilizers. More recently it has shown to be effective in treating depresion, anxiety and PTSD.

We have long known that people afflicted with drug and alcohol abuse have an NAD deficiency. For example, for every molecule of alcohol our liver metabolizes we require an equal amount of NAD+ converting it to NADH.

We know a low NAD/NADH ratio is associated with a craving for drugs and alcohol. The infusion of NAD significantly decreases any withdrawal symptoms and fosters a sense of well being. Dopamine neurons within the mesocorticolimbic circuit (reward circuit) appear to be restored and normalized. By the end of the infusion patients are no longer in withdrawal and report no craving whatsoever, and no desire to use. More recently, the founders of this treatment protocol have begun to offer an oral formulation of NAD that is proving quite effective.

The intensive outpatient detox program is a multi-day program where patients receive a daily intravenous infusion of medications that reduce withdrawal symptoms and cravings. A healthy brain chemistry is gradually restored. Mood, memory, concentration all improve while patients detoxify and slowly heal.

A typical course of treatment lasts 10-15 days. Treatment involves a course of IV therapy. Each day a nurse starts the intravenous infusion of NAD. Additionally, there is an oral supplement program that goes along with the detox program. Withdrawal symptoms improve immediately with the infusion.

The drip is not sedating, nor does it contain opiates or any other addicting substances. The infusion can last between four and eight hours depending on the personalized protocol. Some patients may not tolerate the usual drip rate and require longer sessions. Patients go home at the end of the day.

The Program effectively treats all Opiate, Alcohol and Stimulant Dependence. Some patients who have been on long acting opiates such as buprenorphine or methadone will need a few extra days of detoxification.

Auriculotherapy ~ or auricular therapy, is basically ear acupuncture. Also referred to as auriculoacupuncture, it is a form of alternative medicine based on the idea that the ear is a microsystem which reflects the entire body, represented on the auricle, the outer portion of the ear.

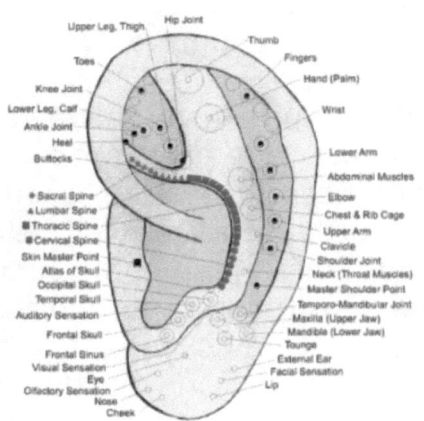

Auricular acupuncture is the stimulation of acupuncture points on the external ear surface for the diagnosis and treatment of health conditions in other areas of the body. The ear is believed to hold a microsystem of the body, consistent with the brain map discoveries of Canadian neuroscientist Wilder Penfield.

Dr. Penfield found that maps of the body exist on the surface, or sensory cortex, of the brain. This same brain map is also projected onto different areas of the body, "microsystems", and in particular precision, onto the ear.

Ear acupuncture has proven to be an efficient method of treating a wide variety of conditions, from headaches and allergies to addictions and pain disorders. Although acupuncture evolved in the context of Asian medicine, the specialty of ear acupuncture was developed in western Europe. It's foundations laid by Dr. Paul Nogier, a neurologist working in France in the 1950's, it was deepened and expanded by Frank Bahr M.D. and physical medicine specialists in Germany over the following decades.

The map on the ear is in form of an inverted fetus with all the fine details of the anatomical, physiological, and emotional body represented. The tissue of the ear is unique and has functions in addition to our sense of 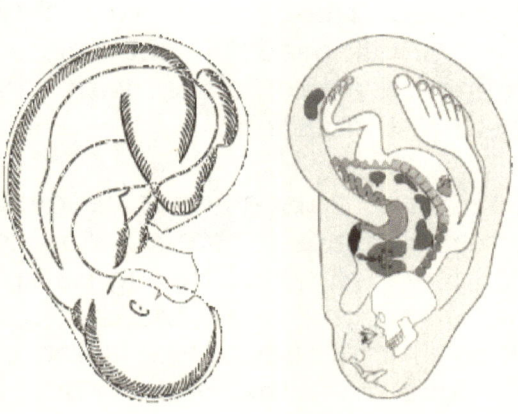 hearing. The ear is the first organ to develop to its full size and become fully functional about eighteen weeks after conception and is one of a few anatomical structures composed of tissue from each of the three primary types (endo, ecto, mesoderm) in the developing embryo.

The earliest use of ear acupuncture, like body acupuncture, dates back to ancient China. Auricular acupuncture as we know it today however is largely the outgrowth of work begun by Dr. Paul Nogier, a neurologist trained in acupuncture. He found that the ear holds all of the acupuncture points of the body plus more detailed physiological and anatomical correspondences and found that stimulation of these points were very effective in alleviating pain and other symptoms.

When an auricular acupuncture point on the ear is "active" it expresses as increased tenderness on stimulation and a higher electrical conductivity. This indicates pathology in the corresponding body tissue or function and makes auricular acupuncture a useful form of assessment of ailments. The texture, colour, skin changes, veins, etc., in different areas of the ear can be indicators of the state of health.

Treatment is performed by needling the respective points on the ear and, if necessary, also on the body. Disposable surgical stainless steel, or gold or silver plated, needles are used. They are inserted only millimeters under the skin. Small 'beads' – metal plated, magnetic, or vaccaria seeds – are often placed with adhesive plaster for longer lasting stimulation.

Children are usually not needled but treated with laser or ear 'beads' instead. All signals induced by ear acupuncture travel through a specific part of the brain, the diencephalon, to the corresponding body parts. The body strictly obeys these commands because they come straight from the brain. Thus ear acupuncture takes advantage of the body's own control center, the brain.

All diseases that can be traced back to a disturbed, but not destroyed, organ function can be treated by ear and body acupuncture: migraine, insomnia, depression, addictions, indigestion, autonomic symptoms, most conditions of pain and inflammation. Some patients feel immediately relieved, others need several days before they notice an improvement. Some people feel as if they were walking on air after treatment, and almost all feel very relaxed.

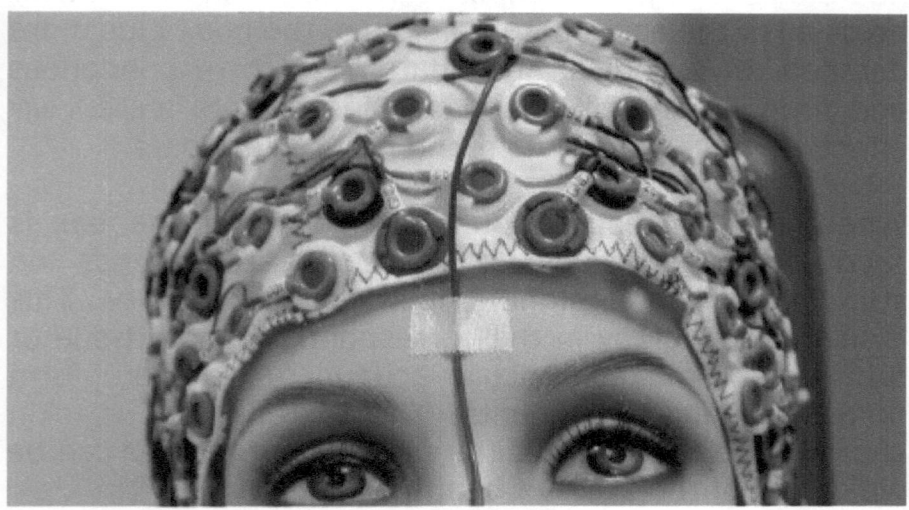

Neurofeedback ~ Neurofeedback is a process by which electroencephalography (EEG) sensors are attached to one's head which allows the brain's activity to be fed back into a computer that displays brain waves in real time. The subject can then interact with her brain waves in order to alter them, directly impacting their frequency.

The procedure is a form of biofeedback, and it has been used for treating a variety of conditions, namely PTSD. Over the past five years, neurofeedback has been gaining traction as a form of alternative treatment at leading recovery and rehab centers. Some addicts claim that it helps with everything from anger to insomnia - key triggers for relapse. The limited science on it is positive but funding for a range of credible controlled studies has been hard to come by.

In essence, neurofeedback can increase or decrease states of arousal – a level of neural activity linked to brain wave frequency. An anxious person would obviously aim for a calmer state (a lower frequency) in a neurofeedback session; someone depressed would seek to create higher frequency and more neural arousal. "It can help keep [addicts] from leaving treatment early," says Matt Morgan, a neurofeedback treatment specialist. While neurofeedback has a forty year history, it is still in its infancy as a treatment form for substance disorders. Morgan says there is "no medication out there with such a wide [therapeutic] use."

About the Authors

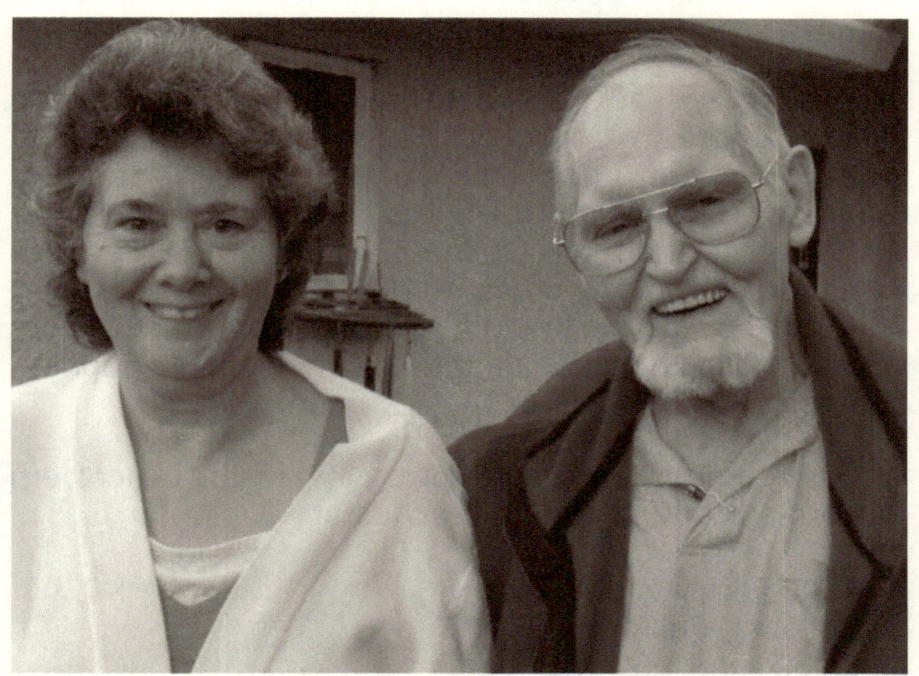

Dr. James V. Potter and Paula M. Potter, husband and wife, are Christian authors, counselors, educators and ordained ministers. Dr. Potter and Paula make their home in Northern California. Prior to moving to California, Dr., and Mrs. Potter served with the Family Ministries School of the University of the Nations, Youth With A Mission (YWAM) in Hawaii; as Associate Pastors with The New Covenant Churches and the Gospel of Salvation Ministries, Hawaii.

They founded the Hawaii Family Care Centers, a network of community-based Christian Counseling Centers in Hawaii, Agape Family Services, Alliance Recovery Services, Advocare Institute and Advocare Publishing Co., dedicated to publishing Christ-centered counseling resources and self-help guides.

Dr. And Paula Potter are Certified Christian Marriage

and Family Therapists, Certified Clinical Pastoral Counselors, Certified Addictions Counselors, and Certified Domestic Violence Specialists.

Dr. Potter was awarded the prestigious Fellow Award by the American College of Forensic Counselors, and is a Diplomate under the American Association of Christian Therapists. Dr. Potter is a member of the World Association for Online Education and is listed in numerous editions of Marquis' Who's Who in America, Who's Who in the World, Who's Who in Religion, Who's Who in Education, in the International Biographical Centre, and In Men of Achievement.

Dr. James Potter, and Paula Potter, MA, reside in northern California USA and can be reached at:

4590 Fairywood Avenue
Redding, California 96003
Email: agapefsi@mail.com

Other Books for Your Enjoyment

Man's soul is priceless -- of value beyond measure -- so valuable that only God's First Beloved Son, Yeshua, could possibly redeem his fallen brothers and sisters. He accomplished this through the Atonement. Soul Care & Soul Cure is an essential tool for pastors, chaplains, counselors, Christian workers, counseling and ministry students and others concerned with the care, cure and transformation of man's soul. It is not only a concise introduction to pastoral care and counseling, it sets forth a plan for integrating the principles of biblical theology and effective psychological practice while holding true to the tenets of each. The need, purpose, goals and objectives of soul care and soul cure are far too often overlooked or misunderstood.

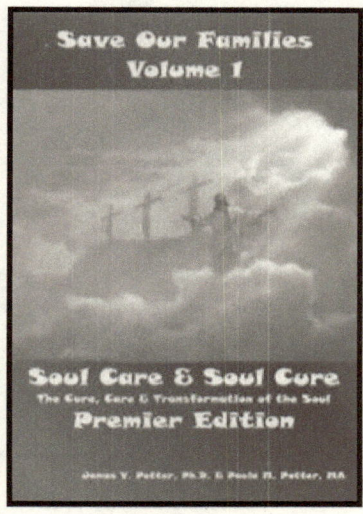

While much has been taught in the church regarding man's need to crucify the flesh and to live and walk in the Spirit, very little has been taught concerning the soul and our responsibility to care for it. Here the authors provide a model for developing church and community based pastoral care ministries -- a model that is both therapeutically efficacious and soul winning.

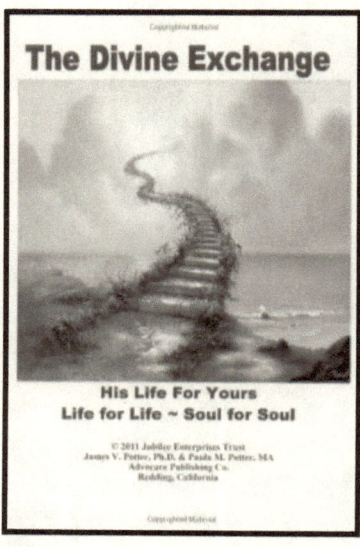

This volume is an account of Yeshua, the Beloved Son of Elohim, who out of unfathonable love came to earth long ago to exchange life for life, soul for soul; to take on humanity, suffer and die in his place, that mankind might be reconciled to Father and enjoy eternal life as a Child of God. When one experiences the Divine Exchange, appropriating every aspect thereof, they will never be the same again. Their flesh will still be subject to decay and death, but their spirit is renewed day by day and their soul transformed. When the exchange is complete, they will be seated with Yeshua in heaven as a co-heir and co-ruler of the universe.

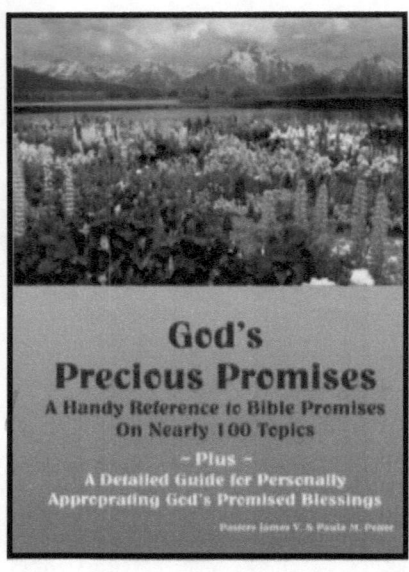

God's
Precious Promises
A Handy Reference to Bible Promises
On Nearly 100 Topics
~ Plus ~
A Detailed Guide for Personally
Appropriating God's Promised Blessings
Pastors James V. & Paula M. Potter

There is an old hymn whose lyrics go, "God is the answer to my every need." In the words of the apostle Peter, "His divine power has given us everything we need for life and godliness . . . He has given us His very great and precious promises, so that through them you may participate in His divine nature and escape the corruption in the world caused by evil desires" (2 Pe 1:2-4). Whatever one's needs, whatever the crisis, God has provided direction and comfort in His Word, if we will but take the time to search through the more than 8,000 and follow the guidance provided us there.

In this collection of Scripture the authors provide you a handy, topically arranged guide for daily living and teach you the keys for unlocking heaven's storehouse and appropriating these promises personally.

Notwithstanding the abundant promises God has provided to fill our ever need, there are two things that can prevent one from realizing these blessings. First, we must use the key that unlocks heaven's storehouse, and second we must resist the Devourer whose aim is to defeat God's children by attacking us, seeking to carry out his plan to steal, destroy and kill (John 10:10).

We are at war, but our battle is not against other humans, it is against principalities and powers of darkness (Eph 6:12). We have been promised that if we resist the Devourer, he must flee, but we must know how to resist, for "the weapons we fight with are not the weapons of the world. On the contrary, they have divine power to demolish strongholds. We demolish arguments and every pretension that sets itself up against the knowledge of God, and we take captive every thought to make it obedient to Christ" (2 Cor 10:3-5). It is a battle we must understand and prepare for to win.

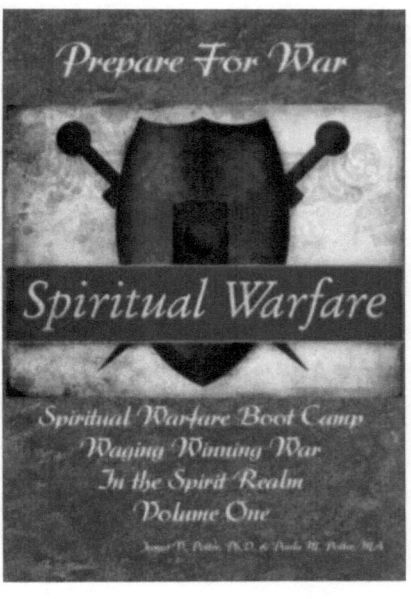

Prepare For War

Spiritual Warfare

Spiritual Warfare Boot Camp
Waging Winning War
In the Spirit Realm
Volume One

James V. Potter, Ph.D. & Paula M. Potter, M.A.

Undertstanding the nature of the battle is one thing, but to wage winning war in the spirit realm we must also know as much as we can about our enemy and his method of warfare. In this second volume on spiritual warfare -- the Synagogue of Satan -- readers are introduced to the panoply of evil beings Satan has under his command, ready to launch an attack at the slightest sign of weakness or vulnerability. This book will prepare you to be victorious in a conflict that you cannot avoid - the battle against demonic forces that oppress and seek to infest, even posses, the souls of men and women.

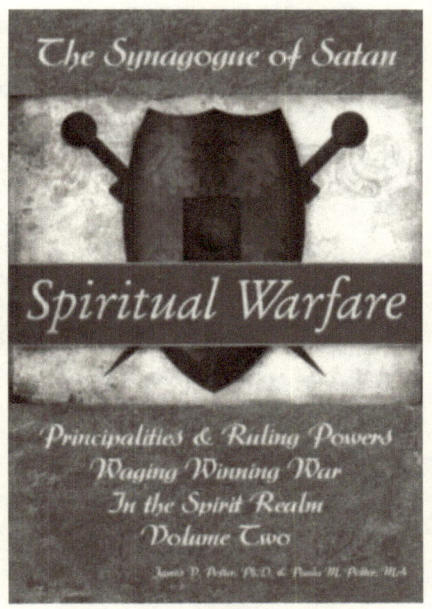

Turning your back on the demons oppressing you may well cost you your possessions, your health, and even your life, for Satan -- their commander -- having been expelled from heaven came to earth with great fury, intent to steal, kill and destroy (John 10:10). But, you need not be one of his victims. Having adequately prepared for this battle, understanding the enemy's identity and strategic battle plan will spell the difference between being victimized or being victorious.

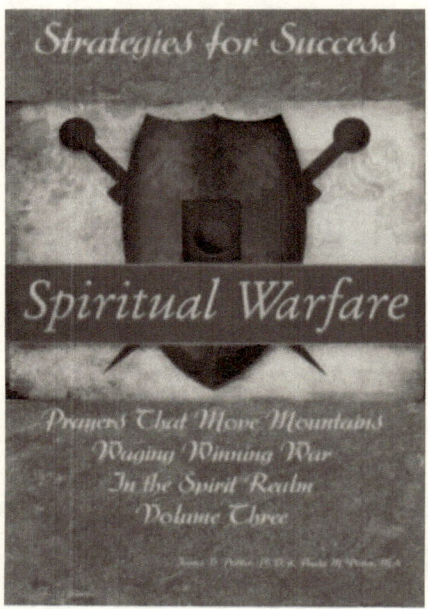

To win in this battle against unseen spirit beings necessitates the use of other-worldly weapons – weapons that can destroy every stronghold, resolve every argument and dispel every pretentious thing. These weapons are at our disposal (2 Cor 10:3-5). But we must know how to use them. In this volume the authors provide strategies for success – prayers that will move spiritual mountains – prayers for the salvation of your children and family members, prayers for your political leaders, religious leaders, coworkers, neighbors and of course, our enemies. But, always remember they are not the real enemy (Eph 6:12).

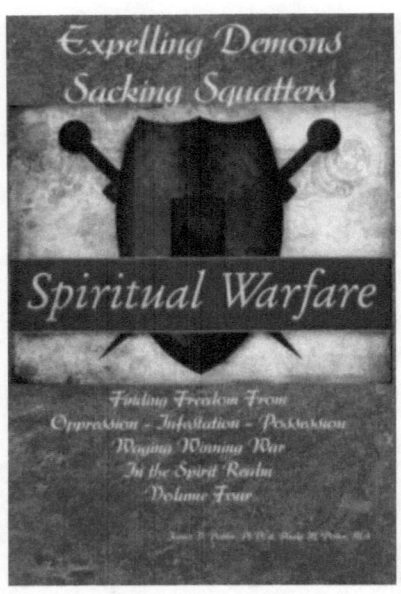

In this, the fourth volume of the series - Waging Winning War in the Spirit Realm - you will gain an understanding of the origin and nature of demons; discover the doorways and windows that allow demons to enter your soul; learn about their legal rights for harassing, infesting - even possessing you; learn the prerequisites for successful deliverance, including preparation for the pastor and the counselee; understand demonic manifestations; and develop skills in deliverance ministry mechanics – all critical for carrying out an effective deliverance. This series, when the information is applied, will make you an effective deliverance minister, equipped to carry out the mandate of Christ Jesus in the Great Commission.

It is imperative that we know the identity of our enemies which the Bible calls evil spirits or demons. Where did the demons come from -- are they the fallen angels, the spirits of deceased evil people, or simply a myth? The Bible has the answer but most read over these difficult to understand sections. However, the mysteries of God are reserved for His children, for His word tells us "It is the glory of God to conceal a thing; but the glory of kings is to search out the matter" (Pro 25:2); And, "God is the God of gods, the Lord of Kings and a revealer of all mysteries" (Dan 2:47). Don't remain in darkness; make it your point to understand the battle between good and evil, light and darkness, so that you may be victorious.

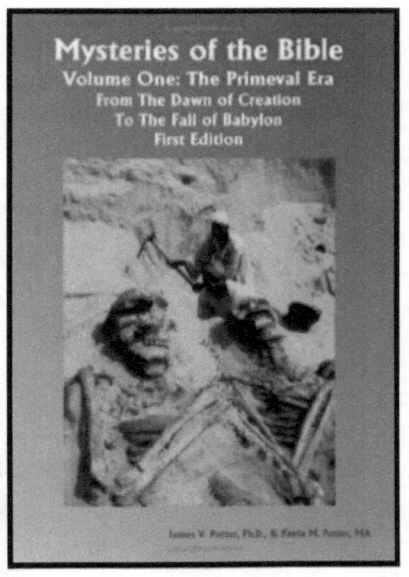

As important as it is to understand the origin of the demons, know the identity of the Devourer and comprehend his battle plan, it is equally important to know the outcome of this battle -- a battle frequently, but erroneously called "The Battle of Armageddon. Jesus said, "As it was in the days of Noah, so it will be at the coming of the Son of Man" (Matt 24:37 & Luke 17:26).

Knowing all we can about the origin of the demons and their present-day assignment, will help us better understand what can be expected in the end-times and how to be prepared. The return of the Nephillm and demons are just the beginning of the changes we can expect as we near the end of time. In Revelation we read, "I saw another angel coming down from heaven having great authority. The earth was lit up by his splendor and he cried out in aloud voice, "She has fallen! She has fallen! **Babel the Great!** She has become a home for demons, a prison for every unclean spirit, a prison for every unclean, hated bird.

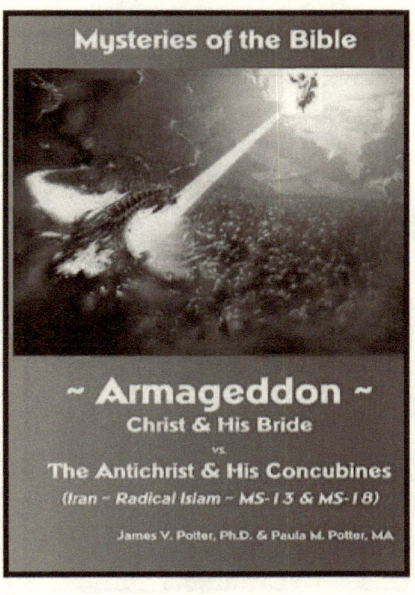

Mysteries of the Bible

~ Armageddon ~
Christ & His Bride
vs.
The Antichrist & His Concubines
(Iran ~ Radical Islam ~ MS-13 & MS-18)

James V. Potter, Ph.D. & Paula M. Potter, MA

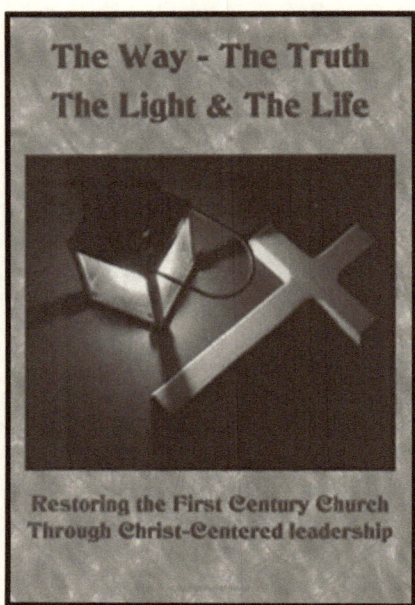

The Way - The Truth
The Light & The Life

Restoring the First Century Church
Through Christ-Centered leadership

"Then I heard another voice out of heaven say: "My people, come out of her! so that you will not share in her sins, so that you will not be infected by her plagues" (Rev 18:1-5). As spiritual Babel falls the saints are called to come out of her but there is still much the church must do to prepare for the return of her Lord. This volume examines what must be done to restore the first-century church. The preeminent requirement will be restoring Christ Centered Leadership within His body - the Bride of Christ - the Church. Discover what we can do now to prepare for this momentous event and learn the prophesied outcome.

As the saints return to the first century model of church and once more embrace Christ-Centered leadership, they can expect the manifestations of signs and wonders that will surpass those of the early church. Speaking of this, Christ said, "Believe me when I say that I am in the Father and the Father is in me; or at least believe on the evidence of the miracles themselves. I tell you the truth, anyone who has faith in me will do what I have been doing. He will do even greater things than these, because I am going to the Father.

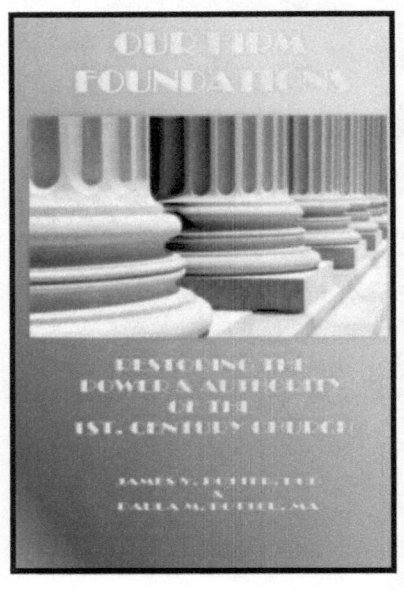

And I will do whatever you ask in my name, so that the Son may bring glory to the Father" (John 14:11-14). In Our Firm Foundations you will discover what we may expect with the power and authority of the first century church are restored. This restored power and authority is the last thing Satan and the demons under his command want to see. Their reaction, was prophesied by John the Revelator, who wrote: "Rejoice, ye heavens, and ye that dwell in them. Woe to the inhabitants of the earth and of the sea! for the devil is come down unto you, having great wrath, because he knoweth that he hath but a short time" (Rev 12:12).

Satan's wrath will be intensified against both the church and the family of man, for could he destroy either, the plan of God – to redeem His children would be thwarted. Recognizing Satan's plan, the authors have written a series of books designed to restore the family of man to the model of the Family of God. They begin by addressing anger, which the apostle Paul says can give the devil a foothold – a doorway into your soul. Yet properly used, anger is a powerful ally. This is why Paul said, **"Be angry, but don't sin** – don't let the sun go down without resolving your anger otherwise you will leave room for the Adversary" (Eph 4:26-27).

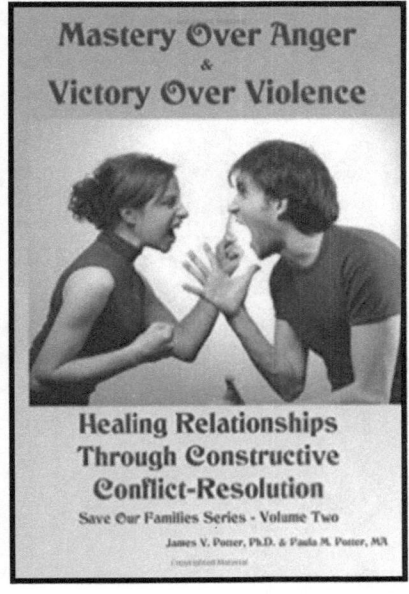

Learning to manage our anger enables one to begin using it to achieve its God-given purpose – to resolve injustices and facilitate healing in our relationships. After learning to manage our anger, there are other skills that are equally important to master.

One of these critical skills is the development and the verbal and behavioral practice of assertiveness. Unlike the aggressive person who seeks to meet their own needs at the expense of others, the passive person who stuffs their feelings, never having their needs met, or the passive-aggressive person who sets out to trigger others' negative behavior, the assertive individual knows how to meet their own needs while simultaneously protecting and helping to meet the needs of others. Assertiveness has been appropriately called the win-win lifestyle. By employing assertive communication and behavior everyone's needs can be met and everyone feels like they are a winner.

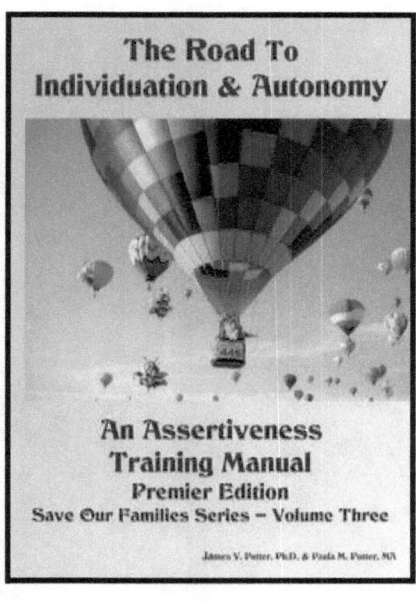

After learning to control anger and embrace an assertive lifestyle, there is another critical change one must work on – conquering codependency. Codependency has rightly been termed the common cold of relationships. Nearly everyone suffers to some degree from codependency. It infects and impacts every member of a family regardless of age, education or gender. Unless it is promptly treated, codependency develops into emotional disorders. Being chronic, progressive and deadly, it is as much a disease as any addiction. Perhaps even worse, it is both a communicable disease and a multigenerational mutation.

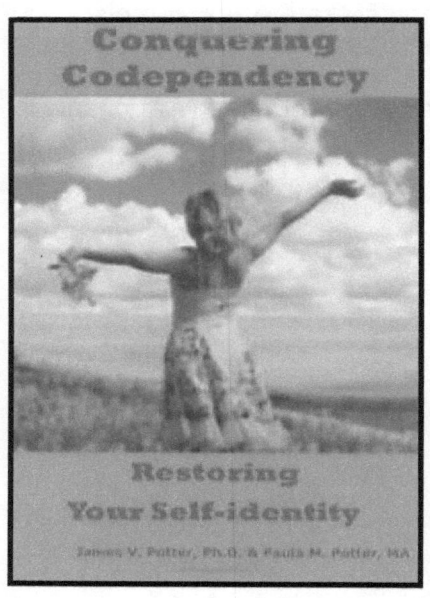

Codependency fractures one's self-image and prevents one from developing a healthy self-identity. Codependents suffer from an identity that stems more from an ego-mass enmeshed with others in their family of origin. While it is a vortex that will engulf the unsuspecting, it can be conquered, leading to a healthful, happy, meaningful life.

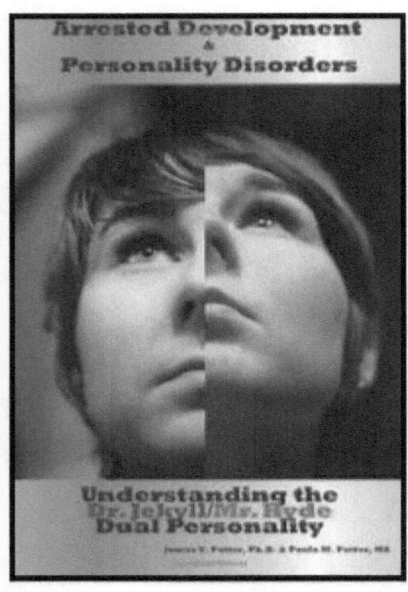

Codependency and the lack of a healthy self-identity are some of the factors that serve to disrupt the progressive human life-span development, and serve as signs of arrested development, leading to mood and personality disorders. The volume incorporates an introduction to the human life-span and its development, an introduction to human attachment bonding, the development tasks of each stage of development and the rites of passage from stage to stage. Thereafter, the volume reveals the origins and manifestations of some of the more common development wounds, explaining how these wounds affect one's temperament, character and personality, often resulting in the development of pseudo, dual and/or chameleonic personalities. Detailed charts depict the impact on an individual's life it developmental tasks are not completed or the rites of passage or go awry. After demonstrating the potential problems, the authors close by introducing exercises that, if followed, will help restore one's personality and heal wounded relationships.

One of the more serious effects of arrested development involves the creation of negative life commandments. A growing body of research suggests that most mental health problems, mood, personality and psychotic disorders are functional in nature, rather than structural. Eminent mental health specialists assert that 75% to 90% of all these problems have their genesis in early-life socio-environmental stress and trauma. This volume addresses the healing of these disorders, employing a biblically based guide for improving one's life commandments popularized as inner-healing or inner-child work

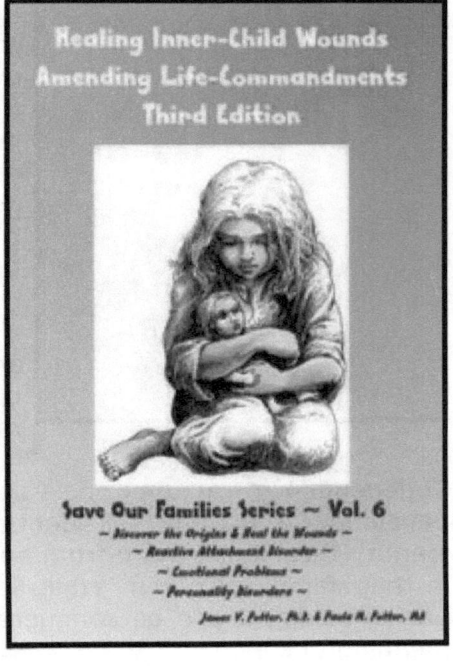

Early-life emotional and spiritual wounds contribute to the onset of substance abuse, dependency, addiction and codependency, but underlying these is a a common thread – toxic shame. Toxic shame exhibits itself in a wide array of fashions, get-ups and garbs. It loves darkness and thrives on secretiveness. It diminishes one's truthfulness, as well as their openness, transparency and humility while simultaneously fueling one's pride and presumptiveness.

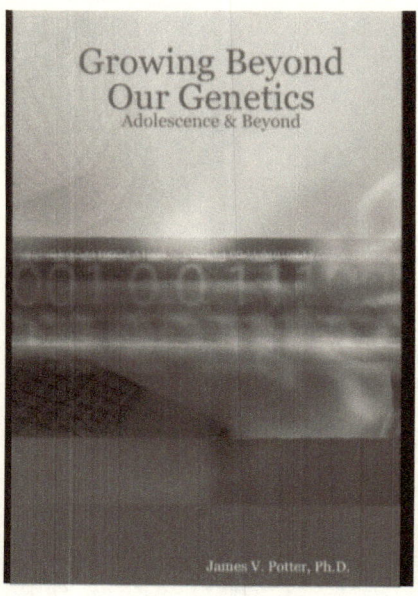

From Toxic Shame

To Freedom

~And The Journey Out~

James V. Potter, Ph.D. & Paula M. Potter, MA

It is the dark, secretive aspects of toxic shame that gives it power – power sufficient to entrap one and imprison them in a dungeon of their own creation. Operating under a cloak of darkness, it evades discovery, identification and examination. Hidden within our subconscious it must be aggressively tracked down and destroyed.

In this volume the authors provide the keys for opening the dungeon to the pathway of freedom and fulfillment, employing the familiar 12-Step model.

Growing Beyond
Our Genetics
Adolescence & Beyond

James V. Potter, Ph.D.

Growing Beyond Our Genetics examines the stage of life we call adolescence that unless navigated properly serves as the origin of Misogynists, Misandrists and Misanthropists, impacting every relationship one strives to create. The authors provide exercises including the development of a Family Timeline and Genogram that promote personhood wholeness, relationship reconciliation, marriage and family relationship restoration and enhancement. These exercises when followed produce true identity metachange and quantum healing. Collectively they manifest the power of the mind-body connection.

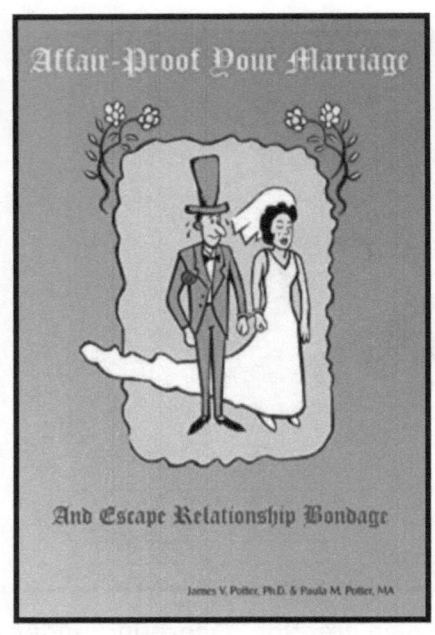

Affair-Proof Your Marriage

And Escape Relationship Bondage

James V. Potter, Ph.D. & Paula M. Potter, MA

These volumes, commencing with Mastery Over Anger & Victory Over Violence through Growing Beyond Our Genetics are collectively a relationship discipleship program used by counsellors and clergy alike to bring healing in marriages and families. The series culminates with this volume that addresses human attachment bonding, which if understood helps couples replace relationship bondage with true bonding, intimacy and oneness.

This groundbreaking marriage enrichment guide is designed to pinpoint issues that negatively impacts human attachment bonding, destroys intimacy and oneness and creates relationship barriers and bondage, resulting in spouses feeling trapped rather than treasured; more like a possession than a prize.

In this guide Dr. Potter and Paula set forth a proven therapeutic approach for breaking through these relationship barriers and replace bondage with bonding, thereby restoring relationship harmony, happiness, spousal intimacy, solidarity and oneness.

Substances of Abuse – is an important companion to the book, Counselling Addicts & Offenders. In this volume you will learn to identify the signs and symptoms of substance abuse and addiction that may be plaguing your marriage, your children, extended family, or friendships. There is an old saying, that Knowledge is Power. Knowing what substance one is addicted to or abusing is the first step toward conducting a successful intervention. In this text – one of the volumes in the "Living Sober; Living Free" series readers are introduced to a proven psychoeducational prevention and treatment program.

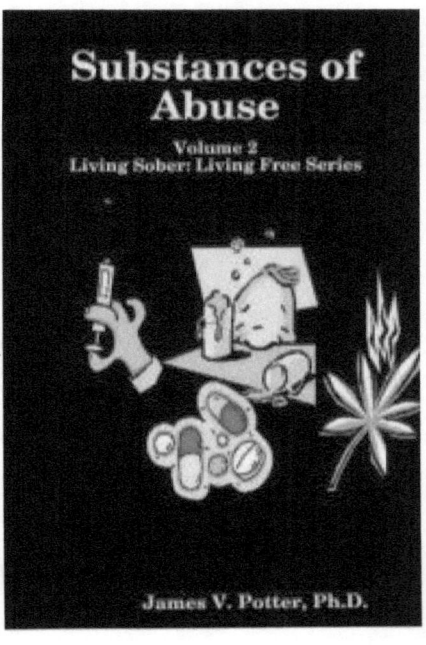

Substances of Abuse

Volume 2
Living Sober: Living Free Series

James V. Potter, Ph.D.

The Living Sober; Living Free program is based on an integrative approach – integrating sound psychological principles and biblical truths. The series is designed for students participating in licensing or certification programs; those seeking college or continuing education credits; substance abuse counsellors; school counsellors; recovery program personnel, nurses, and others seeking information on substance abuse prevention and treatment, including those seeking a self-help approach to living a life free from the bondage of substance abuse, addiction and repetitive criminal justice offences.

The thing that can disrupt marital harmony more than anything else is substance abuse & incarceration with its merry-go-round of arrest, conviction, incarceration, release, re-arrest, etc. If this has plagued your relationship you will be delighted to know that there is a way to get off the merry-go-round! Addicts & Offenders process information very differently than others; their cognitive and affective processes, foundational beliefs, values, attitudes, life-commandments, goals and motivations are different. Understanding this, it is possible to effect meaningful change instead of covering up these issues with band-aids.

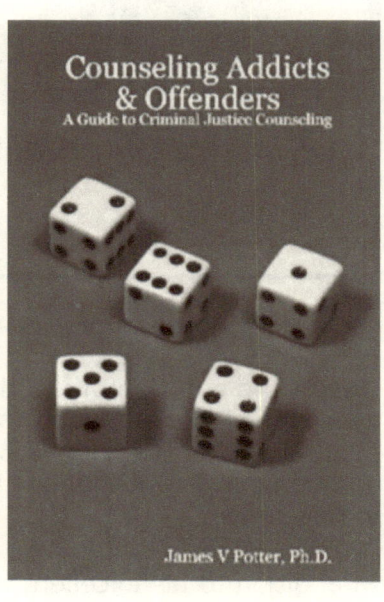

Over the years many have asked about our personal journey of faith. This volume gives you an in-depth glimpse into our personal histories, our marriage and our thirty plus years together, serving the Lord in ministry. We have written it in hopes that our testimony may inspire you to go wherever the Lord calls you and to do whatever He asks of you – even though it may not seem 'reasonable' to your conscious mind. It is our prayer that in reading it you will learn to listen and respond to God's indwelling Spirit, and as you do, to see God work miracles in and through your ministry.

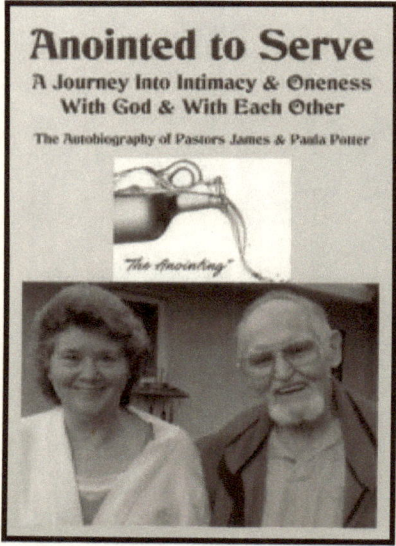

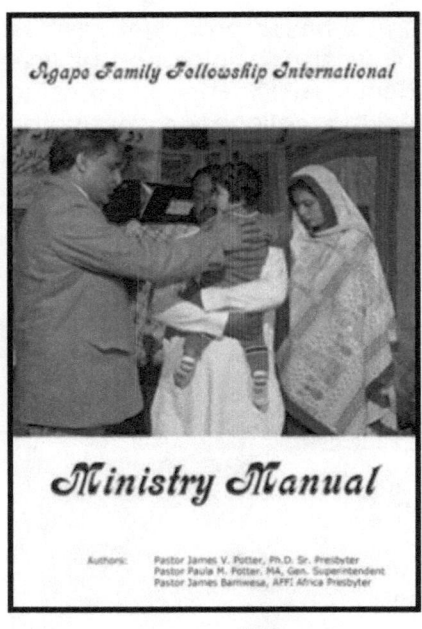

Agape Family Fellowship International

Ministry Manual

Authors: Pastor James V. Potter, Ph.D. Sr. Presbyter
Pastor Paula M. Potter, MA, Gen. Superintendent
Pastor James Bamwesa, AFFI Africa Presbyter

As the ministry that God called us to establish began to grow, many of our affiliate pastors expressed their need to have a guide to govern their work – a guide that would preserve their individual sovereignty yet insure that the fellowships under the banner of Agape Family Fellowship International walk together in harmony, support a common Statement of Faith, Doctrinal Statements and a style of worship that is consistent with the New Testament Apostolic teachings. Since our affiliate pastors and evangelists represent great diversities in backgrounds, cultures and worship styles, we felt it important to provide guidelines that preserved their individual integrity while insuring that heresies do not creep in.

One of the contributors to the development of the Ministry Manual was one of our early affiliate pastors, now the Prelate over the continent of Africa, James Bamwesa. Archbishop Bamwesa has, in addition to his contributions to this manual, authored other volumes in this series.

In addition to his excellent work in the Ministry Manual, Pastor Bamwesa co-authored with Patriarch, Dr. James V. Potter, this excellent Baptismal Manual. This manual has been designed with a dual purpose: 1] to guide pastors in their preparation of baptismal candidates, and 2] to provide new believers a compendium of AFFI's Statement of Faith, Doctrinal Statement, Church organization and style of worship. The manual includes a baptismal vow that is designed to be used when officiating at the baptism and thereafter serve as a reminder to those who are baptized, of their solemn duties.

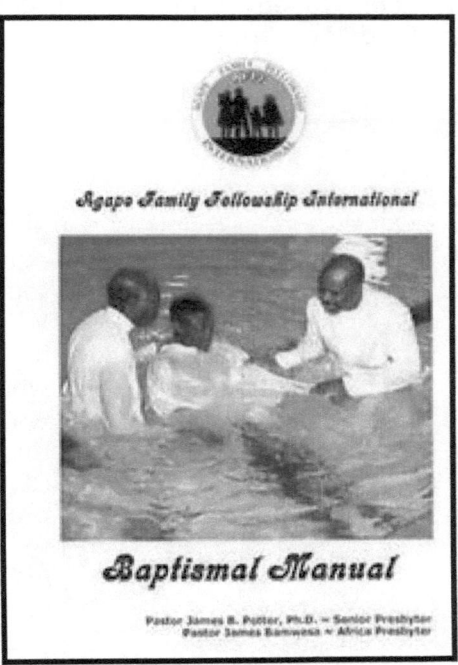

Agape Family Fellowship International

Baptismal Manual

Pastor James B. Potter, Ph.D. ~ Senior Presbyter
Pastor James Bamwesa ~ Africa Presbyter

As the first century church began to mature, the apostles soon realized that while they had been commissioned by the Master to serve as the foundation of the church, their time was becoming consumed to care for logistic details, diminishing their ability to provide spiritual guidance and oversight.

So the Twelve gathered all the disciples together and said, "It would not be right for us to neglect the ministry of the word of God in order to wait on tables. Brothers, choose seven men from among you who are known to be full of the Spirit and wisdom. We will turn this responsibility over to them and will give our attention to prayer and the ministry of the word" (Acts 6:2-4).

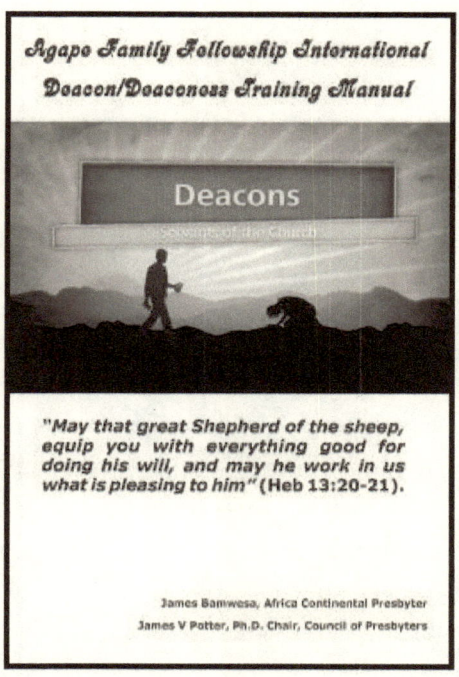

Agape Family Fellowship International
Deacon/Deaconess Training Manual

Deacons
servants of the Church

"May that great Shepherd of the sheep, equip you with everything good for doing his will, and may he work in us what is pleasing to him" (Heb 13:20-21).

James Bamwesa, Africa Continental Presbyter
James V Potter, Ph.D. Chair, Council of Presbyters

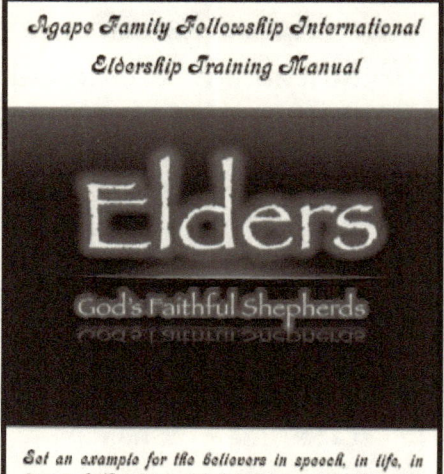

Agape Family Fellowship International
Eldership Training Manual

Elders
God's Faithful Shepherds

Set an example for the believers in speech, in life, in love, in faith and in purity devote yourself to the public reading of Scripture, to preaching and to teaching. Do not neglect your gifts .. given you through a prophetic message when the Body of Elders laid their hands on you (1 Tim 4:12-14).

Pastor James V. Potter, Ph.D.
& Pastor Paula M. Potter, MA

This concept pleased them all and they chose Stephen, Philip, Procorus, Nicanor, Timon, Parmenas and Nicolas who, after they prayed for them and laid hands upon them became the first deacons of the New Testament Church. Today, men and women serve in this capacity. It is our prayer than this training manual authored by Prelate Bamwesa and Doc Potter will aid you in your ministry.

As the ministry of Agape Family Fellowship continued to grow, more and more applications for affiliation were received by individuals who believed they had a calling on their lives to enter the ministry, but had no previous pastoral training or experience.

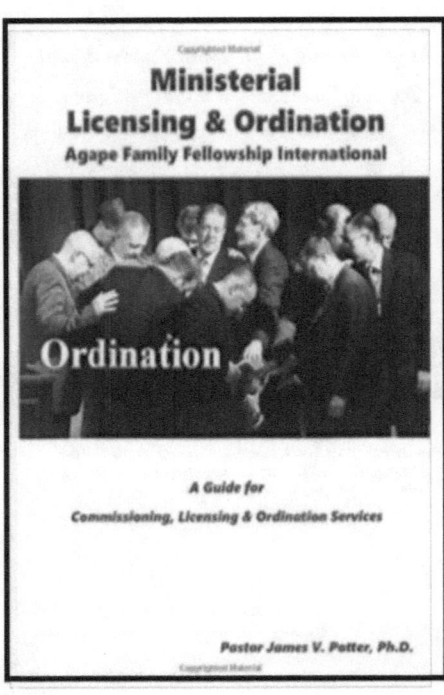

To insure that the call of God on the lives of these men and women is honored, while at the same time insuring that those who represent the ministry are men and women of integrity, have sound doctrine and are free from heresy, this guide was developed. In it we have set forth the biblical guidelines for licensing and ordination as well as providing a model licensing/ordination service.

The initial Ministerial Licensing and Ordination manual, while providing a guideline for those entering the ministry, seemed to fall short in the area of recognizing those who were already qualified, licensed or ordained pastors & evangelists.

To provide for them, and to set in order a program for recognizing and consecrating those already licensed and/or ordained, as well as those individuals being appointed to oversight roles – such as Bishops and Archbishops, this supplementary guide was developed.

While in the future these manuals may be combined into one, at present, they collectively serve as a comprehensive guide for the licensing, ordination and consecration of the leadership of Agape Family Fellowship International. They are also finding favor with many outside of the AFFI ministry.

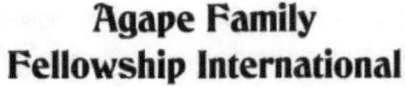

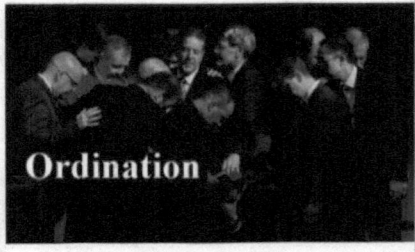

Books by David Honey, Th.D.

Genesis ~ The Story of Man is a verse-by-verse commentary of the story of mankind based on the only authentic source: the Bible. The time period it covers – often referred to as the Primeval Era – commences when our Creator, Father God, said, "Light Be!" And, as the record states, "Light was!" From this beginning, the volume tracks the history of mankind as our ancestors rebelled thereby altering the course of human events and our very solar system itself. It concludes with the call of Abraham through whom God prophetically set in motion a plan to reconcile mankind unto Himself. But the rest of the story waits to be told in Dr. Honey's Genesis – Part Two.

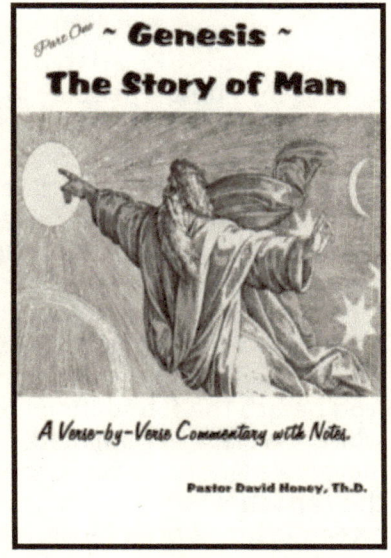

The book "Daniel A Prophecy of Hope" is a verse-by-verse commentary of the Old Testament book of Daniel, that you will want to read and reread. Daniel's prophecies are so diverse you will be challenged by the intriguing imagery that foretold the coming history for the next two thousand, six hundred years! The epic story begins with Nebuchadnezzar - King of Babylon's overthrow of Jerusalem. Daniel and his peers – children of the Israelites' nobility – are taken captive and pressed into service for the king. As the story progresses, Daniel is called upon to interpret the king's dreams – dreams that foretold the future of the Babylonian empire, and the nations that would follow.

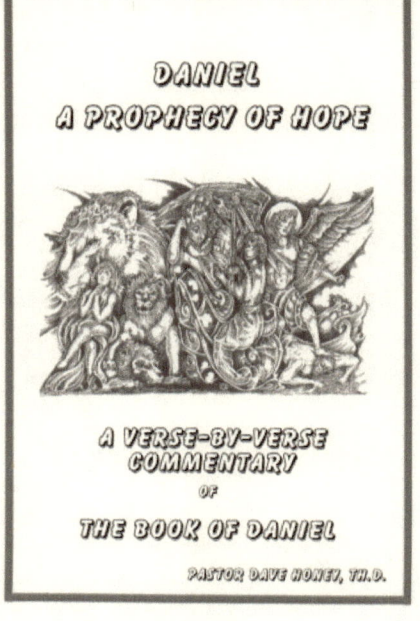

From the rise of Babylon to the fall of Rome, Daniel - guided by Holy Spirit – traces the history of the world that is yet to unfold.

Solved – The Mystery of Revelation – is another Verse-by=Verse commentary by David Honey, Th.D. Pastor David Honey has written "SOLVED! The Mystery of Revelation" to purposely help people better understand the great story of Revelation. The Book of Revelation, written over nineteen centuries ago had our present generation in mind. Although it originates in the ancient past, most of this story still remains to develop in our not too distant future. Conceived in the mind of God before the foundations of the world were established, this incredible story was related to the Apostle John a short time after Jesus Christ visited our world altering it forever.

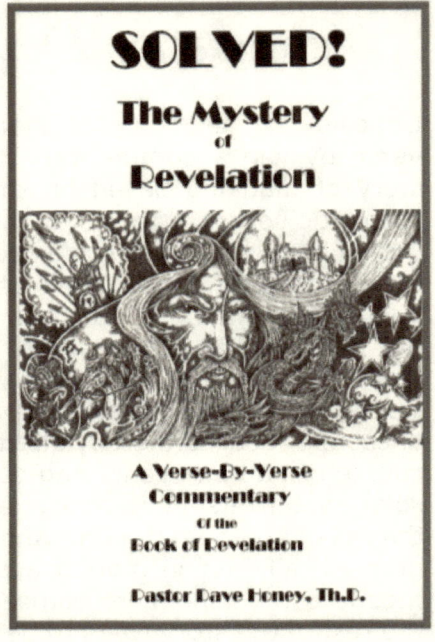

SOLVED!

The Mystery
of
Revelation

A Verse-By-Verse Commentary
of the
Book of Revelation

Pastor Dave Honey, Th.D.

Pastor Honey's Bible Mystery Tours
A Conference Series

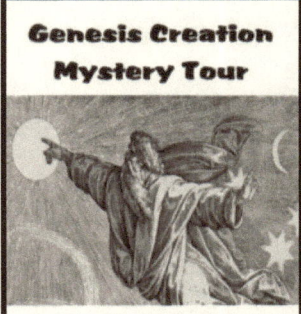

Genesis Creation Mystery Tour

The Biblical Conference Series
Bible Mysteries Revealed

Pastor David Honey, Th.D.

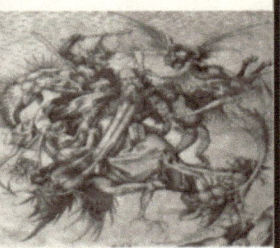

Paranormal Mystery Tour

The Biblical Conference Series
Bible Mysteries Revealed

Pastor David Honey, Th.D.

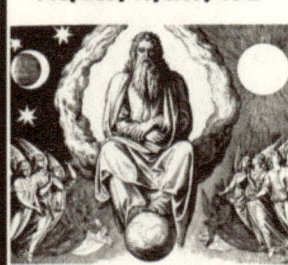

Prophecy Mystery Tour

The Biblical Conference Series
Bible Mysteries Revealed

Pastor David Honey, Th.D.

Angel Mystery Tour

The Biblical Conference Series
Bible Mysteries Revealed

Pastor David Honey, Th.D.

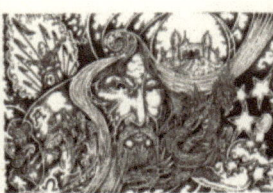

Revelation Mystery Tour

The Biblical Conference Series
Bible Mysteries Revealed

Pastor David Honey, Th.D.

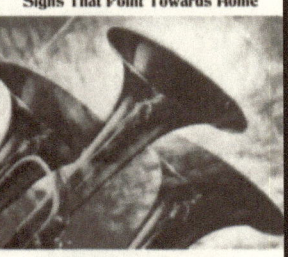

The Coming Trumpet Blast

Signs That Point Towards Home

Biblical Conference Series
Volume Six - Premier Edition
Bible Mysteries Revealed

Pastor David Honey, Th.D.

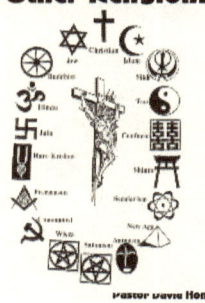

Christianity Cults, The Occult & Other Religions

Pastor David Honey, Th.D

Each of these Biblical Mystery Tour booklets is designed to serve as the text for a two day Equipping the Saints conference. They may be purchased in quantity with quantity discounts, enabling you to provide them to those attending your conference.

www.ingramcontent.com/pod-product-compliance
Lightning Source LLC
Chambersburg PA
CBHW021426170526
45164CB00001B/111